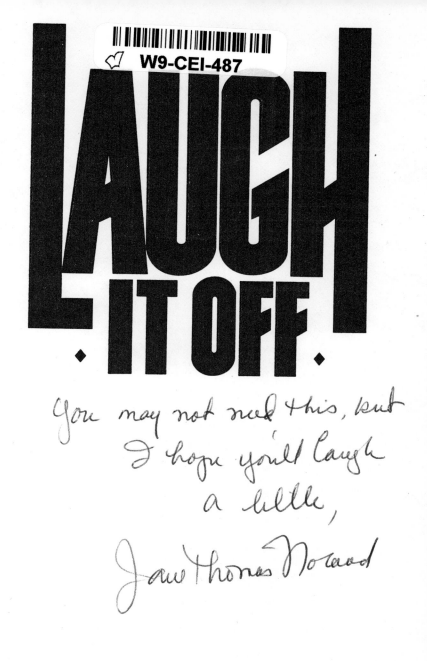

LAUGH IT OFF.

You may not need this, but
I hope you'll laugh
a little,

Jan Thomas Noland

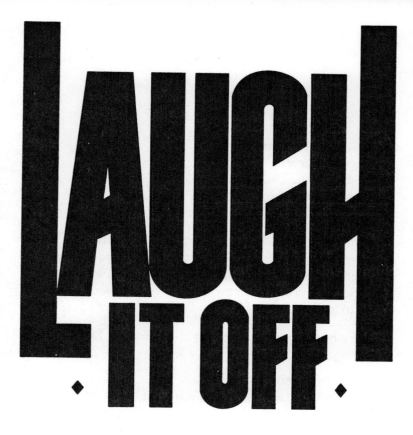

LAUGH IT OFF!

JANE THOMAS NOLAND

Illustrations by Mimi Noland

CompCare®Publishers

2415 Annapolis Lane
Minneapolis, Minnesota 55441

©1991 Jane Thomas Noland
All rights reserved.
Published in the United States
by CompCare Publishers.
ISBN No. 0-89638-249-4

Library of Congress Cataloging-in-Publication Data

Noland, Jane Thomas.
    Laugh it off: new ways to use your sense of humor to
    help you shed pounds / Jane Thomas Noland—Rev. ed.
    p. cm.
    1. Reducing diets. 2. Literary recreations. I. Title.
RM222.2 N65 1991   91-1968
613.2'5—dc20   CIP

Cover design by Jeremy Gale
Illustrations by Mimi Noland and Diane Westby

Inquiries, orders, and catalog requests should be addressed to
CompCare Publishers
2415 Annapolis Lane
Minneapolis, MN 55441
Call toll free 800/328-3330
(Minnesota residents 612/559-4800)

  5   4   3   2   1
95 94 93 92 91

To all those who want to be thinner and who like to laugh

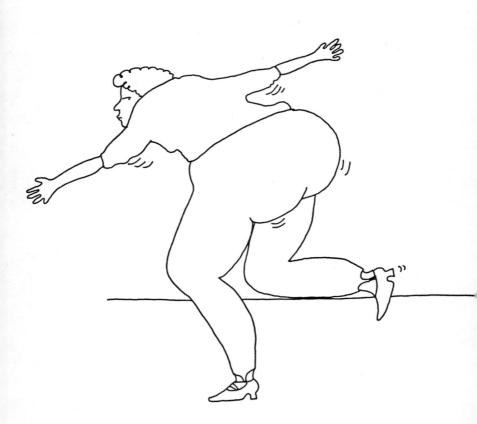

"When you dance, do parts of you go off dancing
by themselves?"

Part I Thinsights: Facing the FAT facts/1

Foreword

In thirty-five years of medical practice, I have observed patients become enthusiastic over many "quick fix" diets. These diets have been touted by "self-made experts," who often have made outlandish, unscientific claims. And too often those who "bought" the "easy, magic" schemes developed unrealistic expectations. Too many of my patients were eventually "rewarded" with disappointment and failure — a few times even with illness.

And still, every six months or so, a new "diet book" or a new dietary supplement or aid seems to appear. Many of these new "diets" develop almost a cult-fad following. Our society gets on and off, on and off, on and off these diet plans and our weight goes up and down, up and down, and up, up, upppp! This method of dieting has been called the yo-yo or the roller coaster. I call it the "Rhythm Method of Girth Control."

The "Rhythm Method" has not, will not, and cannot work. The scientific reasons it cannot work are documented in the dietary advice and literature of the American Heart Association, American Diabetic Association, and the American Cancer Association. These prestigious organizations, along with recognized nutrition experts, espouse the same dietary recommendations: modest calorie restrictions, increased fiber (fruits, vegetables, and grains), a reduction of fat calories to 30 percent or less, and an increase of carbohydrate calories to 55 percent or more. All emphasize exercise as an important adjunct to any weight reduction program.

A number of years ago, amphetamines (often called "speed") were very popular diet pills used as an effective weight reduction "crutch." Unfortunately these "poison pills" resulted in in many physical and mental health problems. The body tissues aged rapidly. Users of amphetamine diet pills often got an unhealthy "high" from these toxic "uppers," and many in our society became unwittingly addicted.

In the past twenty years, medical science has identified a class of chemicals that is revolutionizing weight reduction efforts. These chemicals are safe, nontoxic, easy to take — and can be refilled without a prescription! These "medications" are the endorphins, chemicals that each of us makes in our own "internal pharmacy" — the brain. It's all "in the head!"

The endorphins are related to synthetic morphine, but are estimated to be 2,000 percent more potent than injectable morphine. The endorphins, called our "inner uppers," have many healthy physiologic properties that get us "high on life." The endorphins can suppress body and mind pain, ease body and mind tensions, enhance immune function, afford a mental "euphoria," and SUPPRESS THE APPETITE!

There are many healthy pleasures that can raise the level of these "inner uppers." They are raised by exercise — by connecting with community, friends, and relatives, — by selective pleasant sensations of touch, sight, sound, smell — by *imaging* pos"I"tively — and by LAUGHTER AND HAPPY THOUGHTS!

At last Jane Noland has put the puzzle together. Jane has developed for us a weight-loss book we can all go to often to get that special boost — that dose of healthy pleasure — that prescription to "laugh for the health of it!" Here's a "diet book" that will never be "recalled" by the FDA, a "diet book" that rewards instead of punishes, a "diet book" that will help us all "lighten up" — and lighten up!

Laugh It Off is a book about losing weight that can "add days to your life and life to your days"!

Yes, the magic "inner uppers" are manufactured in the head. They can even be "faked up" by pretending — by faking a laugh or a smile.

I give my patients a laughter prescription that reads: "Stand in front of the mirror, look at yourself, and belly-laugh for fifteen seconds twice a day." Some patients will say, "You have to show me something to make me laugh." I tell them, "That's why you do it in front of the mirror."

Perhaps we should be laughing more at our foibles and follies when it comes to weight reduction. Perhaps a major solution for weight reduction is to raise the endorphins. Imagine that! Laughter may be ha-ha-ha-hazardous to your waist!

Dale L. Anderson, M.D.

Dr. Anderson is a board certified, Mayo Clinic trained general surgeon and a board certified emergency physician with over thirty years of health care experience. He has a clinical practice in the orthopedic department of the Park Nicollet Medical Center in Minneapolis, the fifth largest multi-specialty clinic in the country. He is also medical director of SHAPE, Inc., a division of the clinic that promotes wellness and conducts programs and seminars throughout the country. Dr. Anderson is known nationally as a speaker and health "edu-tainer."

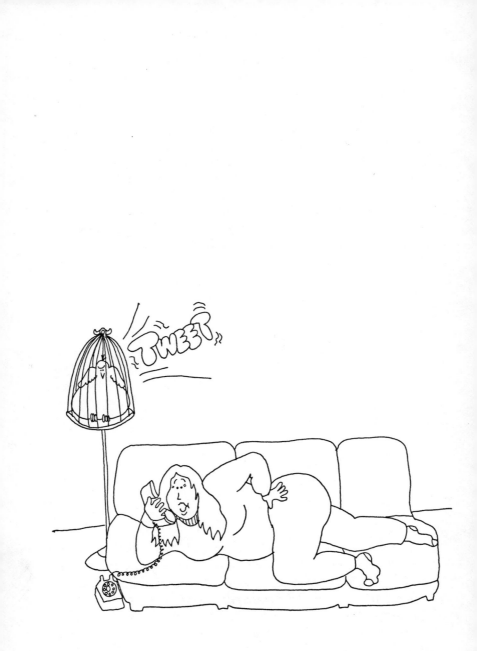

"I can't understand it. I eat like a bird."

Author's Preface

The ideas capsulized in this book — some new, some borrowed, some assimilated from years of experience in weight-loss groups — are thoughts to get thin by. Along with this collective wisdom, you'll find Humor Strategies to keep you looking at the light side as you learn to define your own kind of humor and apply it to your first priority — your Project ME.

Losing weight does not have to be a time of gloom and martyrdom. This affirmative, anti-FAT workbook can help you find the joy of positive thinning. No matter what weight-loss program you're on — whether you're losing with a group or a clinic or on your own — put laughter to work for you. Cultivate your own good sense of humor — and let it help you *Laugh It Off.*

Think of your extra pounds as a burden, like a heavy piece of furniture you and a couple of others are attempting to move — an oak buffet, for instance. What happens if you get the giggles? Your muscles relax and you drop the buffet. (Watch your toes!)

The burden of extra weight is a lot like that piece of furniture. Laughter can help you drop that weight you're carrying as part of you. My conviction, after gaining and losing hundreds of pounds over the years and watching others do the same, is that we chronic pound-adders and pound-shedders have overlooked one very obvious aid to weight loss: a healthy, built-in sense of humor.

How does humor and laughter affect weight loss? Count the ways!

Laughter helps alter our endorphin levels. More and more recent evidence links laughter and positive thoughts with a healthy body. Some theories now are relating certain brain-generated, endogenous opiates — peptides, called endorphins — to appetite suppression. So, it seems that laughing is one of the things we can do to generate these "inner uppers" that may make us less hungry!

Laughter is exercise. We've known for a long time that a hearty, whole-person laugh is great exercise for our body systems, including cardiovascular and respiratory. Observations of writers like Dr. James Walsh *(Laughter and Health)* have borne this out.

Laughter heals. Norman Cousins in his classic *Anatomy of an Illness* described how he used old Marx Brothers films and other visual funnies to help himself heal from a serious illness. (Those endorphins again?) In the foreword to Allen Klein's *The Healing Power of Humor,* Dr. Carl O. Simonton says that sientific research is now bringing us new understanding of the old saying, 'Laughter is the best medicine.'

If laughter can help us heal from disease, it can also help us heal from the dis-ease of too much weight.

Laughter is a stress-reliever. So many of us are stress eaters. Like other animals who have shown increased foraging behavior under stress, we, too, find ourselves foraging in the kitchen or at the nearest fast-food place when we're tense, facing deadlines, trapped in stress-producing situations.

In *Dr. Lendon Smith's Low-Stress Diet,* Dr. Smith says that "stress can lead to overweight in susceptible people," that "obesity is a sign that the body is experiencing stress." Although we are all different and there is no "snappy, universal answer" to weight loss, his makes-sense theory is that if we eat appropriately, exercise moderately, lead a sane lifestyle, and alleviate stresses, the symptom of obesity will disappear.

What better way to reduce stress than through humor and laughter!

Allen Klein in *The Healing Power of Humor* says, "Humor can diffuse our stressful events. It relieves built-up tension and pops the cork off such things as fear, hostility, rage, and anger."

Laughter helps us "disconnect" from our obsessions with weight. Through humor, we objectify our all-consuming problem of being all-consuming — and of *"having to* lose weight."* And that objectivity helps to free us so we can! It's hard to maintain the balance of just what your body needs when you're compulsive or obsessive about the shoulds and oughts of your "diet." Thoughts about food whirl constantly in your head: "Do I dare eat THAT?" "How can I can get rid of the calories consumed in yesterday's binge?" "What food goodies am I going to reward myself with, once I get thin?" If your weight control (or out-of-control) has become an obsession, learn to lighten up — with laughter.

Laughter helps us break through our denial about being overweight. The only way to take that First Step (of the Twelve Steps of Overeaters Anonymous) and admit powerlessness over food is to acknowledge the problem. Humor softens the harsh reality of our own overweight, so that we can brave the mirror to look at ourselves honestly. If we overeaters, like alcoholics or compulsive gamblers, can see the absurdities of our food compulsions, laughter becomes a liberator. Once we've overcome the denial, humor helps us get rid of unhelpful feelings of guilt and take measures to change.

Laughter helps us avoid discouragement and depression about our overweight. Discouragement can derail the most fervent and faithful weight-loss program. Humor helps us be realistic about goals — how fast the pounds can leave us and how many we can lose — a day at a time.

We'd be out-of-touch Pollyannas to believe that all of life is fun and laughter, that laughter is always appropriate. It isn't. But if we can learn to be open to the humor around us — the irony, the exaggerations, the comparisons, the delightful twists of language — and celebrate it with laughter, we'll discover a technique that can actually help us pare down to our thin selves.

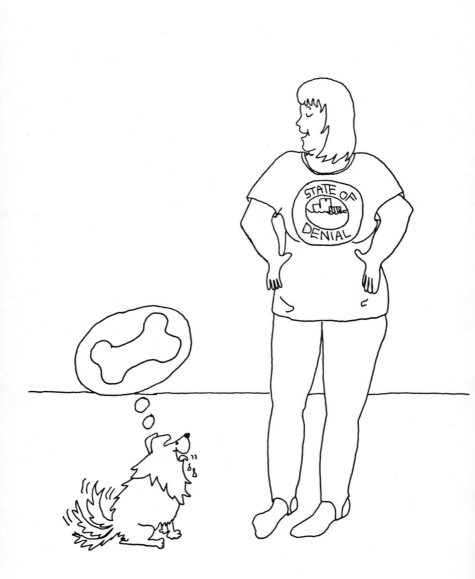

"I'm not fat. I just have BIG BONES."

Part One

Thinsights:
Facing the FAT facts

The sayings, songs,
and thoughts herein
can guide us all
from thick
to thin.

The Good News Is . . .

The hope is that by taking a long look at our extra poundage, we will realize that our overweight is, indeed, an inescapable fact.

No leaning against the wall while standing on the scale. No balancing a toe on the ground. None of that quick stepping on and off before the flickering indicator has time to zoom up and land on a true reading. We all know the tricks.

Write down your real, honest weight. No more ducking the truth. Extra pounds can be bad *bad news* for your health and your self-esteem — affecting your life and the lives of people close to you.

Just recognizing and accepting that fact can be the first move toward doing something about it.

Now the *good news*. I, too, can become thin and healthy. We've all known ex-heavies who have turned their lives around and are now one hundred, fifty, forty, twenty pounds lighter. Listen to these thinner winners. Each has an idea or two to contribute to my personal Project Thin.

I Hate FAT

In building up a good case of dislike for FAT, I must remember that it is not I, ME, MYSELF that I dislike, but only the extra weight that keeps me a prisoner in my own fat cells.

I hate what FAT does to me. FAT:

tightens my shoes,

launches my buttons,

peekaboos my seams,

gives me varicose veins and back problems and blisters on my inner thighs,

makes my zippers — or my pantyhose — crawl downward — usually while I'm hurrying for a bus or carrying a cafeteria tray or on my way to a podium,

makes my belt buckles face down,

leaves strap-furrows in my shoulders and sock-dents below my knees.

FAT brings me ILL health, ILL feelings, an ILL nature, and ILLusions.

I hate FAT. Enough to do something about it NOW. Not tomorrow morning or after my sister's wedding or my friend's catered dinner party. Not after I've polished off the rest of that bag of bakery items I just bought. (I can always feed them to the dog or the kids next door.)

NOW.

The Blame Game

I must beware, while working up a useful anti-FAT anger, not to give in to that common copout: blaming. We're inclined to blame our weight on everyone and everything, to shift the responsibility away from ourselves.

I blame (check one or more):

☐ My parents for my body type.

☐ My husband for getting home from work so late that I eat multiple suppers — one with kids, one with spouse, one with the dog (with whom I also share the table scraps).

☐ My wife. Ditto.

☐ A weak back. A sore knee. A sprung tendon. Any impairment, however slight, that keeps me potatoed out on the couch.

☐ My job. "I'm under all that pressure at work — no wonder I eat!" or "It's all those fancy lunches with clients!" or "I work around food all the time" or "I'm stuck at my desk — spreading." Add your own job-related excuse here:

_____

☐ That fast food place, for establishing itself within walking distance of home.

☐ The world economy for driving up the prices of good-for-you foods. Getting into global excuse-making, I can blame heads of state, legislators, drouth, locusts, and the IRS.

☐ My favorite uncle, who introduced me, at the impressionable age of two, to the sugary, addictive pleasures of the soda fountain, thus launching me on a lifelong course of equating food with good times.

☐ The PTSA for asking me to contribute to the annual bake sale. (How can a responsible parent refuse?)

- [ ] The phone company for installing a stretch cord that extends to the refrigerator.
- [ ] My housemate/soulmate for cooking all the wrong things.
- [ ] The Girl Scouts for selling those "but it's only once a year" cookies.
- [ ] The high school band for pushing candy to earn money for uniforms.
- [ ] My homework because "I always eat when I study."
- [ ] Henry Ford for popularizing the automobile, so we don't walk around much anymore.
- [ ] The Persians for discovering how to process sugar cane juice into solid sugar.
- [ ] My friends for inviting me to dinner.
- [ ] My son for insisting that I accompany him to the hockey banquet.
- [ ] My kids, who douse me with guilt when I am not being a "good mother who bakes" after-school crisps and gooeys.
- [ ] My mother for *being* a "good mother who bakes" — who supplied *me* with the above.
- [ ] My "good grandmother who bakes," who taught my "good mother who bakes," who taught *me* . . .etc., etc., ad rotundum.

What other obscure cause can I find to blame my fat on:
I blame:

_____

_____

_____

_____

Reluctant conclusion:
I alone am responsible for my own overweight.
I deserve to be thin.
I can choose to change.

The HOWs of OW (Overweight)

An honest ditty

We tend to relate
our own overweight
to wherefore's and why's multitudinous.
But that's misconstruing.
It's all our own doing.
Quite simply,
we put too much food in us.

FAT gets in my way
I can't see the ankles for the knees

Some specifics:

Do I need convincing that I am an overweight thin person, a thin person gone FAT?

Oh, no. I'm convinced all right. I have a scale, after all, and a full-length mirror (but is it full-width?) and a picture window that reflects at night. There I am, in all my overblown amplitude. I cannot escape the largeness of me.

If I refuse to step on the scale or be enlightened by reflections, there is always the ultimate moment of reckoning — the occasional, painful, necessary clothes-shopping trip.

But do I realize just how much my overweight gets in my way? Probably not. We FAT thin people are such fantasists. Most of us would just as soon not face our FAT, in a mirror or any other way. We are still dreaming that a doctor or a nutritionist or a wizard of some sort will come up with a magic weight-losing scheme that will carry us effortlessly to our thin goal. We even hope for some cozy little illness — very minor, of course — to help pare us down.

Sometimes we have to force ourselves to look at our FATness before we can bestir us to find our thin selves.

How, exactly, does my extra weight affect my social and personal life, my job or career, my physical activity, my economic status, my health (emotional, physical and mental), even my spiritual well-being?

Is my compulsive overeating and/or the consequence of overeating — overweight — negatively and consistently affecting one or more aspects of my life?

The answer, if we will just let it sink in, is that FAT does make a difference, a B-I-I-I-G difference!

How about my physical activity? Even in everyday household chores, FAT gets in my way. I think about it before I climb on a stepladder, hang a window shade, plug in a floor lamp, run up to the attic or down to the basement laundry, clean my topmost cupboards. If I stand too long, my feet hurt. If I sit too long, I feel guilty. If I go to the bed in order to forget the whole FAT problem, I don't get anything done. I huff sometimes, from the mildest exertion.

My sporting life is seriously hampered. In sports which thinner people do well, from Ping-pong to racquetball, I end up in the handicapped-by-FAT league.

A. I turn purple tying my bowling shoes.
B. I wouldn't be caught red sunning or swimming in a bikini (or in a pair of balloon shorts or a granny one-piecer, either).
C. On the tennis court, my stamina runs out before the court time.
D. My cross-country skis submarine a good four inches below the snow's surface, while the rest of the ski group skims by. If I fall down, which is likely, I make a permanent angel in the snow.
E. I can't mount a horse without either ruining some-body's station wagon fender or requiring a three-person leg (and seat) up. Once I'm atop, the horse complains.
F. I don't run. I don't jog. I slog (that is an incredibly slow jog).
G. Whatever I do, I am aware of my extra warm-up suit of adipose tissue (a storehouse for plain old FAT) jouncing and tugging.

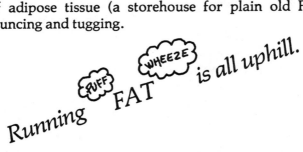

Running {PUFF} FAT {WHEEZE} is all uphill.

More serious than being assigned to the inactive file is the possibility of ill health and early death. To name a few of the problems which have been linked with overweight: varicose veins, hypertension, heart attacks, hemorrhoids, cancer, diabetes, digestive disease, kidney disease, gall-bladder disease, back trouble, arthritis, skin irritations, difficulties in pregnancy and childbirth. Not funny.

When it comes to my career/job/profession, I can pretend that my extra weight doesn't interfere — but in spite of denials by certain employers and personnel departments, FAT counts — against me, especially if I am a woman.

What employer, looking for someone to represent the organization, when given the choice between an attractive, thin, fashionable, self-assured woman and a dumpy, unsure one wouldn't choose the former? What employer wouldn't prefer a dish to a platter? (My apologies to sensitive feminists, but to a long-overweight non-dish, being viewed as a dish is not all bad.)

By the time I reach the hiring line, I already may have met FAT discrimination in that college admissions department which passed me by for an equally qualified, but thinner, candidate.

No matter how unjust we feel it is, our civilization associates FAT with sloth, passivity, stagnation, sluggishness, dullness, laziness, lethargy, torpor and non-achievement. Such judgments are unfair, and many of us heavies become superachievers and excellent workers to counteract the stereotype of FAT-and-lazy or FAT-and-dull.

Certain professions still are limited to thins; I cannot become a FAT jockey, a FAT airline pilot or steward or stewardess. Branches of the military also have weight-in-proportion-to-height limitations.

If I'm heavy, I won't even bother to apply for a job as a fashion model, a trapeze artist, a professional basketball player, a shoe salesperson (I don't balance well on those little footstools), a spa attendant, a tennis or golf pro, a high-rise construction worker, a high-rise window washer, a supper club cocktail waitress, a ballet dancer, or a PR person. Even vast Wagnerian opera singers are out of vogue, now that it has been well demonstrated that a barrel for a voice chamber is not a prerequisite for distinguished performance at the Met.

Overweight doctors, nurses and others in the health professions contend with a double dose of scorn, because of the assumption that anyone who *knows* about being thin and healthy ought to *be* thin and healthy. When it comes to careers, we FAT thin people have a choice.

1. We can take up our banners and climb on our soapboxes (if they'll hold us) to harangue against the thin world's insensitivity to FAT. We then become examples of FAT non-stereotypes.
2. We can change ourselves into *thin* thin persons — thins who have a real understanding for the problems of the overweight.

One overweight's conclusion: It is a whole lot easier to put down your fork than to transform the attitudes of an entire civilization. While it may be comforting to know that your chunky great-great-grandchild might not be teased by the thin kids, there is no way to wring that kind of promise from the future. Let's think about us, now, and how we fit into our world today.

Economically, FAT — and what it takes grocery-wise to maintain it — puts a bulge in the budget. Just one dieter in a family has been known to cut food expenditures drastically. Then there are the side outlays for extra doctor bills, reducing salons, exercise machines, shoes (FATS seem to wear out shoes faster), more clothes in more sizes, counseling services (for depressions related to overweight), higher life insurance premiums, sturdier furniture.

Ecologically, if I and all other overweight American adults would diet off our estimated 2.3 billion excess pounds and keep them off, the energy saved each year thereafter — as we maintain our normal weight — would be 97 trillion BTU's or more than enough to cover the annual residential energy consumption of New York City or meet the needs of four other major cities — Boston, Chicago, San Francisco and Washington.

This idea was presented by Dr. Bruce Hannon, a statistician and energy researcher, and Dr. Timothy

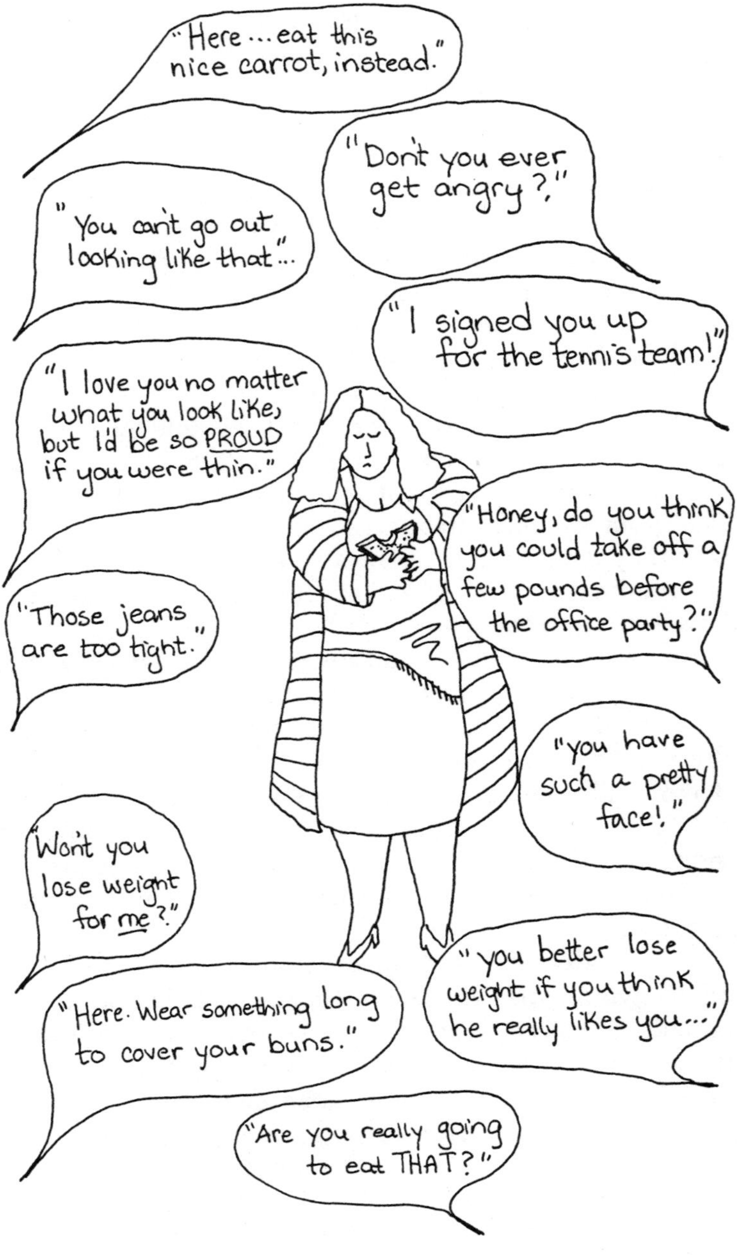
"Here... eat this nice carrot, instead."
"Don't you ever get angry?"
"You can't go out looking like that"...
"I signed you up for the tennis team!"
"I love you no matter what you look like, but I'd be so PROUD if you were thin."
"Honey, do you think you could take off a few pounds before the office party?"
"Those jeans are too tight."
"you have such a pretty face!"
"Won't you lose weight for me?"
"you better lose weight if you think he really likes you..."
"Here. Wear something long to cover your buns."
"Are you really going to eat THAT?"

Lohman, a nutritionist and physical fitness researcher at the University of Illinois, in an article in the *American Journal of Public Health.* This is based on calculations which indicate that it takes 25 to 28 British Thermal Units (BTUs) to produce a calorie of food, including all the energy used in raising and feeding animals, fishing, planting, cultivating, harvesting, processing, transporting, marketing, storing and cooking. Yearly savings in calories would be 3.4 trillion* if the former overweights maintained their lighter weights.

What could *I* personally, save in BTUs if I cut my caloric intake? (Get out the calculator.)

Emotionally, FAT is crippling. Just what my overweight does to my regard for myself is enough to keep me in a perpetual downdraft. (If you think FAT is unrelated to emotions, see *FAT and feelings.* Also observe how you feel when you cut your food intake, not for a day or two, but over a long enough period of time to see your life patterns changing. You may be stunned at the feelings that float to the surface — angers, resentments, hurts and fears that you have been stifling in pillows of FAT and tranquilizing with food.)

Spiritually, FAT may be cheating me out of strengths that are available to me. Am I blaming God for my FAT? God gave us perfectly good bodies. We, ourselves, have distorted them with FAT. I can't blame a Higher Power for spooning food into me.

The following sample situations, derived from the FATalogues of some of those who are now on their way to being thin, can offer us a lesson in realism, that wide-angle mirror we need in order to face up to our FAT facts.

Have you ever:
1. Sat on the sidelines of a volleyball game because you didn't want to raise your arms up and show your flabby midriff?
2. Blurred your eyes as you passed store windows, so

---

*Jean Mayer and Johanna Dwyer, "Dieting Slims Not Only You, but U.S. Energy Needs, Too," *The Minneapolis Star*, Wed., Feb. 14, 1979.

you couldn't see your dumpy reflection?

3. Not stepped on the scale for months at a time?

4. Lied about your weight on your driver's license, thinking, "They'll never know because I don't *look* as if I weigh that much!"?

4. Stayed home from your child's third-grade play because you could not fit in third-grade-sized chairs? (When you get up, you take them with you — affixed to your behind!)

5. Hidden empty cereal bowls under the bed, only to have the dog dig them out and give away your secret stash?

6. Taken a behind-the-scenes job in the mailroom or the kitchen or the book stacks because you didn't want to meet people?

7. Been offered a behind-the-scenes job in the mailroom or the kitchen or the book stacks because *your employer* didn't want you to meet people?

8. Made excuses to avoid going to your high school reunion because nobody would know you, now that you've added 47 pounds (plus a few years)?

9. Torn into the grocery bags looking for a particular food item *as* the bags are being loaded into your car? (I mean, you are still in the pickup area!)

10. Opened a box of snacks in your grocery cart, then closed it up again before you checked it out, so the checkout girl wouldn't know you'd been nibbling? (Or worse yet, had to explain to the checkout girl that you opened it yourself, since she was about to send it back apologetically for another box?)

11. Had a bed break under you?

12. Had a chair — a perfectly good 20th century chair — turn to kindling beneath you?

13. Dieted successfully all day long, only to blow the whole thing by overeating in the evening?

14. Turned down a sleighride (hayride) because if you fell off you couldn't possibly catch up?

15. Turned down an invitation to go rollerskating because you would mash anybody you ran into, and

FAT pays a greens fee

I yelled, so all could hear me, "FORE,"
And then my bulged anterior
Eclipsed the ball. My Wilson "1"
Had vanished like the setting sun
Behind the curved rim of my midriff.
(All who noticed caught me mid-whiff.)
I have learned, though I can tee it
I can't swing if I can't see it.

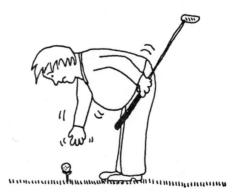

if you fell down you would never get up?

16. Discovered that your thighs didn't fit under your typewriter table?

17. Had sore feet all the time you were on them (and some of the time you weren't)?

18. Fallen off a ski tow and not been able to untangle yourself, forcing the operators to stop the machinery and assist you?

19. Avoided beaches and pools?

20. Worn a long-sleeved, navy blue raincoat, even in 103-degree weather?

21. Been drawn, like a magnet, into a bakery or soda fountain when you had no previous intention of stopping?

22. Been envious — to the point of dislike — of a thin person?

23. Felt your shoes fill up with snow or soak through with rain because you couldn't find any boots to fit you?

24. Gotten up every morning for _____ years (fill in your own number) with the proclamation, "This is the day I am going to get serious about my diet"? By the time 10 a.m. rolls around, you have decided that **tomorrow** is the day.

25. Tried every new diet you ever heard about, even the ones you *knew* were crazy?

26. Returned an armload of slacks to a salesperson with the comment, "They aren't quite right," when the truth was you couldn't get them up over your knees?

27. Felt so defiant after some member of your family asked, "How's the weight coming?" that you went directly to the refrigerator?

28. Disguised your chewing noises on the telephone?

29. Pulled back from your mate's romantic advances because you were embarassed about your body?

30. Huffed when you ran? Or been afraid to run at all?

31. "Outgrown" downhill skiing, skating, other sports you used to do regularly?

32. Gone fishing by yourself (because the boat would

swamp with any more weight than yours alone)?

33. Been unable to see over the bow of the boat when you were in the stern?
34. Gotten your FAT fingers stuck in a bowling ball?
35. Been uninvited to play on the employees' baseball team?
36. Taken up two seats on a carnival ferris wheel?
37. Noticed that other ferris-wheel riders look nervous when they see you buying a ticket?
38. Discovered that your social life is limited to pen pals and crank calls?
39. Developed an extra seam in the lower abdomen because your lap overlaps?
40. Been so embarrassed to eat in public that you refuse to dine out? Or if you do, you keep your overcoat on?
41. Been passed over as a concert or theater companion because your friends blush when the people behind you can't see?
42. Not been invited to go to the beach because others know that you would be humiliated to bare your body?
43. Found it hard to find a mate?
44. If you already have a mate, worried about keeping him/her?
45. Cut down the length of your stride by several inches because you are hampered by the lowered crotch on your pantyhose?
46. Neglected to wear an automobile seat belt because adjusting it to fasten around you was a) a bother or b) impossible?
47. Avoided buying clothes because you didn't want the humiliation of the fitting-room fits?
48. Gotten up in the middle of the night to finish off a favorite food item that you knew was waiting impatiently for you in the kitchen?
49. Had your wrap skirt unwrap in public?
50. Been depressed about being overweight?

Twenty telling questions

I have looked at the uncomfortable specifics of just how FAT gets in my way. By this inductive process, I am ready at this moment, _____ (fill in the date and year), to face these twenty general questions. I don't have to answer yes to all twenty to prove to myself that I am, indeed, a compulsive overeater. A nod of recognition over any one of these may tell me that I have an eating problem. A yes to five or more means that I probably am a first-class overstuffer.

1. Do I eat for other reasons besides hunger — because I am anxious, bored, guilty, nervous, worn out, hurt, lonely, angry, joyful, relieved?
2. Am I embarrassed about my overeating?
3. Do I hide my overeating from others — engage in solo nibbling, visit food drive-ins alone, eat before or after family mealtimes?
4. Do I avoid new situations, new challenges — such as a new job — because I feel that my extra pounds or my eating habits are handicaps?
5. Do I avoid meeting people because I feel self-conscious about their intitial reaction to my overweight?
6. Do I sometimes (or often) lie about my weight — about how much I weigh now or about how much I have lost on a diet?
7. Is my negative attitude about my overweight dragging down my total self-image, how I feel about non-weight-related aspects of myself?
8. Do I sometimes, suddenly and unpredictably, give in to a food temptation I was sure I could resist?
9. Do I have "binge foods" — certain foods that I can't

seem to get enough of? (These may not always be the same foods during a person's lifetime; foods change their appeal from time to time.)

10. Do I find myself thinking a lot about food, referring to food in my conversations, reading cook books or magazine articles about food?
11. Do I get panicky when I think I am going to be without food, stranded somewhere where I can't get to it or locked up without it?
12. Do I fortify myself against such a foodless emergency by carrying food around with me — in my car, in my pockets, in my purse?
13. Have I tried diet after diet with minimal success?
14. Have I dieted successfully, only to seesaw back up to where I was when I started?
15. Has my overweight had a negative effect on my business, career, profession, school life?
16. Has my overweight had a negative effect on my social life?
17. Has my overweight gotten in the way of developing — or keeping — an intimate personal relationship, such as a marriage?
18. Has my overweight affected my health?
19. Am I afraid that being overweight may shorten my life?
20. Have I become so discouraged about my weight that I want to give up trying to lose?

Overweight equals OW.

FAT words

COLOSSAL PORTLY PUTSY
MONUMENTAL WHALE-LIKE
WEIGHTY AMPLITUDINOUS
BLOCKY WHOPPING MACRO-
SCOPIC OVERSIZE DUMPY PLUMP
BIG MASSIVE LUBBERLY GROSS
CHUBBY HEAVY BULKY BLUBBERY
LARGE HUGE CORPULENT TUBBY MEA-
TY CHUNKY LUMPY STOCKY GIGANTIC
FLESHY ELEPHANTINE GIANT ENORMOUS
CAPACIOUS MONSTROUS PUDGY BEEFY
PODGY GARGANTUAN OBESE MAMMOTH
TURGID IMMENSE ROTUND AMPLE STOUT
OUTSIZE MOUNTAINOUS VAST JUMBO
GORBELLIED BROAD OVERBLOWN
OVERSTUFFED FUBSY OVERFED HOG-
LIKE PIGGISH TITANIC SWOLLEN
PUFFY SQUARE MEGALITHIC
PADDED UPHOLSTERED ROLY-
POLY ROUND GOG-LIKE
MAGOG-LIKE POT-BELLIED

Can you think of more?

Thin words

willowy
slight
spindly
thin
trim
slim
sylphlike
sticklike
twiggy
lissome
skinny
lithe
wiry

If I take time to notice, there "I" am in all of them. I notice, too, that our vocabularies are stuffed with FAT words. In fact, there are many more plump words than skinny ones. FAT is unusual, out-of-the-ordinary, abnormal, noticeable. FAT is meat for gossip or the low-volume aside. We need all those weighty words to talk about FAT and FATTIES.

Thin is too normal to talk about. Thin is no fun to discuss — unless you have recently become it. *Then* it's fun, all right!

X out the FAT words — FAT X's, one for each FAT word. (Go ahead. This is an anti-FAT workbook.) Imagine that you are Xing out your Xtra, and the Xcesses that made you that way.

Then think of thin words. Concentrate on thin words.

I will find my place in the middle of thIn.

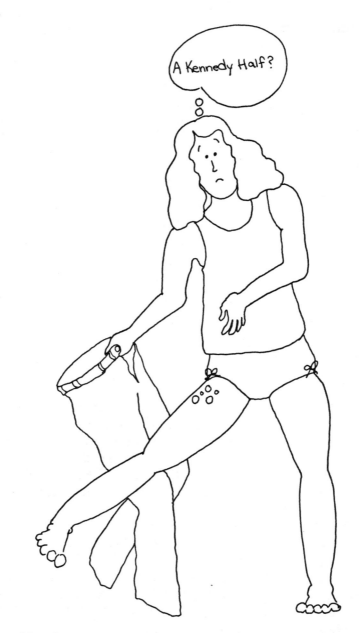

You know your jeans are too tight when your pocket change is embossed on your thighs.

Getting thin — with good reason.

If I could drop a pound for every good reason I have for losing weight, I'd be a broomstick.

Do I need extra fuel to launch myself into less space — as a thin person?

Do I need more ammunition for the Great American FATfight?

Do I need a few more "whereas's" for my personal Declaration of Independence from FAT?

I will list here the tangible effects of my compulsive overeating, effects that I face every day. Check those appropriate to your sex, style of living and degree of overweight. I will be free from:

☐ Sagging sofas
☐ Sagging bed springs
☐ Sagging knees
☐ A sagging bosom
☐ Sagging spirits
☐ An over-awareness of gravity
☐ Sticky fingers
☐ Sticky typewriter keys
☐ A sticky steering wheel
☐ A sticky TV channel selector
☐ A belt dent
☐ Sock dents on my calves
☐ Shoulder-strap furrows
☐ Creases around my upper middle
☐ Creases around my lower middle
☐ Creases under my chin
☐ Crumbs in the bed
☐ Crumbs in the car
☐ Crumbs in my pocket
☐ Crumbs in my cleavage

- ☐ Big furniture-repair bills
- ☐ Big pants
- ☐ Big skirts
- ☐ Big underwear
- ☐ Big blazers
- ☐ A closetful of clothes in four sizes
- ☐ Sore feet
- ☐ Toed-in pleats on trousers that had to be "eased"

Add your own good reasons:

_____

_____

_____

_____

_____

_____

_____

_____

_____

_____

_____

_____

_____

_____

_____

_____

_____

FAT

WADDLES, BOUNCES, ROLLS (a sailor's gait on dry land), HUFFS, PUFFS, LUFFS (baggy clothes in the wind), SIGHS, DRAGS, AMBLES, LOLLS, MEANDERS, SAUNTERS, SLUMPS, SLOPS, DAWDLES, LANGUISHES, LOAFS, SLOUCHES, SAGS, LAGS, HANGS, LOITERS, IDLES, DROOPS, RESTS, TIRES, MOPES, AVOIDS, STANDS AND WATCHES, SITS A LOT

Add some of your own: _____

_____

_____

_____

_____

_____

THIN

skims, soars, glides, hikes, hustles, dances, climbs, flies, runs, jogs, races, rushes, performs, achieves, acts, reaches, springs, bounds, darts, sprints, moves a lot

Add some of your own: _____

_____

_____

_____

_____

_____

Humor Strategy

In order to make humor work for you, first define what makes you laugh.

Is it watching slapstick, pratfalls, a chase on the screen? (Certain Pink Panther movies reduce me to jelly. So does the car chase through the fields in that old classic flim, *The Flimflam Man.*) Video rentals can be an endless source of humor.

Is it a cartoon style? Find a favorite cartoonist, like George Booth or Gary Larson. (In our family, we count on Jerry Van Amerongen to double us up with his bizarre goings-on in "The Neighborhood.")

Is it playing with words and sounds? Puns? Punch lines? Double meanings? Spoonerisms? (I, for one, never cease to get feeble with laughter over "chew in the back of the purch" spoonerisms — those switched-around beginning consonants — as in the silly ditty that begins "I once had a fog named Dido — I've had him since he puz a wup." Or even better are the spoonerisms that happen by mistake in the rush-and-tumble of everyday talk. If you are one of those whose inner circuits seemed to be crossed often enough to produce spoonerisms — relax and laugh about it!)

Do you laugh at the irony of role reversals? For example, your six-year-old plays your own discipline back at you as she chides you for not eating the bread crusts "that make your hair curly — so you save a lot of money on permanents!"

How about fantasy? People pretending to be animals? Or animals pretending to be people? Imagine yourself as a playful animal who seems to laugh, hugely and visibly — like a dolphin. Feel yourself as a dolphin moving weightlessly in the sea. Enjoy that sense of weightlessness. Then imagine yourself laughing and moving effortlessly as a thinner person.

Find *your* brand of humor. Discover what makes you laugh. And use it to help you get thin!

I wear my FAT as . . .

I am not a FAT person. I am a thin person encased in a hampering FAT. We were not designed to be FAT. The human body is made to thin specifications. It is not supposed to be as wide — or almost as wide — as it is high. For all of us who carry extra pounds around, that is just what they are — "extra" pounds.

I will not honor FAT by considering it part of my real, God-designed self. I will regard FAT as a temporary departure from normality, some excess layers built up through my own unwise eating habits. Anything I built myself I can also tear down.

FAT is not a part of the real me.

By realizing how I wear my FAT, maybe I can find ways to get rid of it.

How do I wear my excess poundage? **Check one or more of the following:**

- ☐ As a Superman or Wonder Woman cape
- ☐ As a pillow
- ☐ As an armor
- ☐ As a burden
- ☐ As an old overcoat
- ☐ As a clown suit
- ☐ As a weapon
- ☐ As a shroud
- ☐ As any other costume (specify) _____

_____

_____

_____

_____

_____

_____

_____

_____

I wear my FAT as a Superperson cape

I wear my FAT heroically, like some kind of magical cape — the kind worn by a Batperson or a Superperson or a cartoon wizard or a galactic good guy. I am a FAT Merlin, a Mary Poppin'-her-seams.

I am the strong and mighty one. I am Superdad, Mightymom, Supergrandmother, Superfriend, Superboss, Wonderperson. I am superconscientious about responsibilities — my own and other people's.

I am the helper-outer, the jump-in-and-rescuer, the person always in control, the organizer. I take everybody's problems on my own mighty (FAT) shoulders, whether I am asked to or not, while I ignore an important problem of my own — taking care of myself.

I wear my FAT with epic grandeur. Someone could write a book about my rescue operations, as I try to be all things to all people.

I bustle and accomplish and achieve, but bustling is exhausting for a heavyweight. (I would never in a million years of overeating let on that I am tired out from mere FAT.) I am the undefeated, the pillar, the harbor, the haven, the home. And I will probably drop dead someday if I don't get rid of my FAT Superperson cape.

My schedule is as heavy as I am. My feet hurt as I race from commitment to commitment. Oh, how the world needs Mighty Me (and how I need to be needed!).

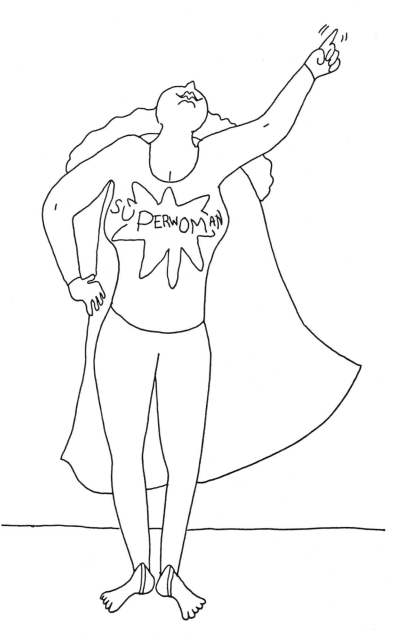

I am the strong and mighty one

I wear my FAT as a pillow

I come equipped with a FAT pillow, a built-in safety device to cushion me from crashes of all kinds — from unrequited love to mail fraud. I count on my FAT pillow for security. I sit on it, lie on it, kneel on it, walk on it, hide my head in it.

For a long time now I have been plumping up my FAT pillow, which now has me thoroughly sound-proofed, people-proofed and emotion-proofed. No matter what kind of a blow or nasty surprise fate may throw my way, I can be assured that my FAT pillow will protect me from stubbing my toes or skinning my shins on unpleasant reality.

Even though the hubbub of humansville seems far off sometimes, and my own responses come through muffled, I continue to feather my FAT pillow. After all, it *is* safe behind it. And I am such a supersensitive type that I need cushioning.

A few simple test questions will tell me if I wear my FAT as a pillow (unless I already know it). What would I do first if:

1. I overheard somebody say something negative about me?
   - ☐ Write a huffy note
   - ☐ Cry
   - ☐ Eat
   - ☐ Kick a wall
2. I learned about an upcoming divorce in the family?
   - ☐ Recommend a counselor
   - ☐ Eat
   - ☐ Rush to tell the rest of the family
   - ☐ Demand that they patch it up
3. My neighbor's Dachshund bit me — imagine the injustice — while I was sharing my lunch with him?
   - ☐ Paddle the dog (not hard)
   - ☐ Eat (the rest of my lunch)

☐ Lapse into hurting silence
☐ Shrug it off and go after a Band-Aid

4. My children's pranks brought on the wrath of the local law officer?
   ☐ Rant about ungrateful offspring
   ☐ Lock them up
   ☐ Eat
   ☐ Invite the officer in for coffee and sensibility

5. Nobody told me about an office get-together?
   ☐ Resign
   ☐ Blow up at the trainee
   ☐ Send a bitter office-wide memo
   ☐ Eat

If my first reaction to these situations was to eat, then I can be quite sure I wear my FAT as a pillow.
To go about unplumping my FAT pillow, I will:

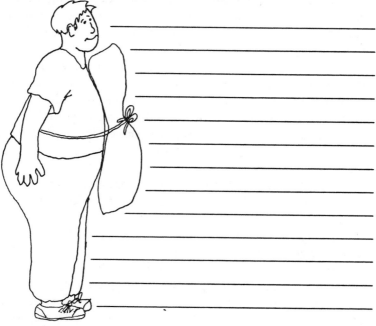

My fat pillow will protect me

I wear my FAT as an armor

I might just as well be clattering around in hinged boiler plate and chain mail, since I wear my FAT as an armor. What am I protecting myself against? An overinvolvement with life and other living human beings? The very thing that I want the most I am the most fearful about — especially now that I am hung with all of these unwished-for pounds.

Although I yearn for the beauties of intimacy, I either don't know how to go about finding it, or I am afraid of the responsibilities that go with it. My FAT is, both figuratively and physically, a way of keeping people at a chubby arm's length.

Have you ever met a heavy person embittered over a love dissolved, a marriage gone sour, a job dead-ended after a large investment of self? That particular heavy is — no way! — going to risk a similar disaster. Or have you known a young man or woman still depending on the childhood family for protection and identity, someone who desires an individual personhood more than anything in the world, but doesn't know where to begin? When these non-riskers — or burned riskers who have decided that the risk isn't worth a repetition of the pain — become heavier than ever, they feel even more vulnerable. And FAT becomes an armor. (If I am an armored tank whose non-risking is based more on defiance than on fears, I may be wearing my FAT not only as an armor, but also as a weapon.)

I will listen to myself for clue statements like these:

"You go ahead. I have a lot of things to do at home." (Eating is one of them.)

"I really don't want to meet her. She's not my type." (Are you worried that you may not be *her* type?)

"I don't need to clutter up my life with new people or new things to do. It's complicated enough already!"

My considered conclusion: Armor is uncomfortable. If I am going to make the most of living, I need to step out of it. I especially need to get rid of that double-thickness breastplate I wear over my heart. I may think I am strong and self-sufficient, but I am actually a prisoner in my own defenses.

If overeating and overweight are my armor, I need to clank up my visor and peer out and see what, precisely, I am arming myself against. I need to know that softness can be strength, that admitting vulnerability can be the first step toward constructive disarmament.

I will take the following specific steps to relegate my armor to the scrap heap. (Plan your own armor-chucking program here.)

_____

_____

_____

_____

_____

_____

_____

_____

_____

_____

_____

_____

Armor is uncomfortable

33

I wear my FAT as a burden

Heavy, heavy hangs on my body and in my spirit. I am a down person, which is not astonishing since gravity is yanking me in that direction. Not only does gravity drag me down, but I pull everyone around me down. too. I wear my FAT as a burden, a gunnysack weighty with "poor me" feelings. Fate has played a wicked trick on me by saddling me with this big body, and I take out my unhappiness on anyone whose life touches mine. Since I am weighed down with miseries, no one else deserves to be happy, either.

Whereas other FATfolk withdraw and suffer in silence, I suffer out loud. Listen to me moan:

"I need a ride to the doctor this afternoon. I just can't take a bus." (Unsaid, but understood: **I'm too FAT to swing myself up the bus stairs, and the bus line is too far from the doctor's office for me to walk.**)

"Do you mind bringing me that accounts file?" (Unsaid, but understood: **I'm too FAT to get up and bend over the files to find it.**)

"You know I don't like to go to the beach. I get so hot." (Unsaid, but understood: **You'd get hot too, if you wore a coat to the beach, I'm too unsightly to unbutton it to let in a little breeze.**

"If I'm doing the cooking, we're going to eat right here. I can't handle a picnic." (Unsaid, but understood: **Imagine me, hauling my bulk and a picnic basket through a field somewhere. Or trying to cook over a campfire. How ridiculous!**)

"I know the dog pants a lot, and is out of shape from living in an apartment. But who's going to walk him?" (Unsaid, but understood: Not me! It's all I can do to get up and down the stairs to let him out in his pen. I pant, too.)

"They sure don't make shoes the way they used to! These wore out in two months. I'm going to write the company and get my money back." (Unsaid, and probably *not* understood by the shoe company: Under my heavy tread, shoe leather might as well be tissue paper. But it's still the company's fault for making shoes that don't hold up under heavyweights.)

Since I'm "not like other people," I talk a lot about doctors who puzzle over me and my ailments.

I ask favors. I lean on others as messengers, fetchers and substitutes. I have bad posture. I meld with sofas. The lines pressed around my mouth have the downward curve of walrus tusks. I have a satchel of troubles that I'm willing to dump on anyone foolish or kind-hearted enough to listen. I am the living antithesis of the "jolly FAT."

Where do I start to change? By gathering up the gloom I have poured out all over everyone within earshot and admitting that *my* weight is *my* problem. If I listen to myself, I will hear how I "share" my personal burden with the whole put-upon world.

If I am powerless over food, I need Power from somewhere . . . preferably Higher. I need to know that I CAN change, that I am not unique and unable to lose. Am I hanging onto my burden in order to hang onto others?

What will I do to lay my burden down? _____

_____

_____

_____

_____

_____

I wear my FAT as an old overcoat

My FAT is an old overcoat, a thrift-shop special, which gives me the seedy, down-at-the-heels look of a true foodaholic.

My FAT is an excuse to be sloppy. I can't possibly look decent anyway when I'm so FAT, so why try?

I don't think much of myself — even of the inner, thinner me. I pretend that I "don't really care," that "it's too late to do anything about it."

I'm a defeatist. I give up easily. I don't deserve to be thin. And since I am heavy, I don't deserve to act, dress, behave, live like a thin person. The good, thin life is so far out of my reach that I will probably strain something if I go after it.

Other people say they care about me, but I don't believe them. How could anyone possibly care about bulging, overblown me? My clothes wrinkle. So do my one-time waistline and my fleshy back.

I am not a lot of fun to be with. In fact, I'm a real bore — for everyone, including my draggy, dowdy self.

I cover myself casually with separates. The bigger the better, because as I enlarge — as I undoubtedly will — I need room to expand. I sneer, defensively, at others' preoccupation with self-appearance and such earthly trappings as clothes.

With attitudes like these, there is nowhere to go but up (on the scale, that is).

But honesty is the best persuader. Of course I care. I will not be swamped by my FAT overcoat. Reshaping myself is such a huge challenge that I will see my own encouraging self-betterment almost immediately. I can start by saying out loud, "I deserve to be thin." Not just once, but enough times so that it sinks in and I begin to believe it. If I can't find a handy private place to say it aloud (the world is running short of handy private places), I will at least say it in a stage whisper loud enough for *me* to hear. Just mouthing the words does not seem to work as well. I need the sound of my voice to startle me into accepting the idea. Yes, sir. Yes, ma'am. I *do* deserve to be thin!

Since I have been lax about grooming, have "let myself go," as they say, it takes a very small effort to effect a big change. If I can't get rid of my old overcoat overnight, I can at least send it to the cleaners. To my surprise, I find that I spend less time worrying about how I look since I have begun to feel less down-and-out FAT and more respectable. I see now that I, with my negative self-indulgence, was really more preoccupied with appearance than those thinner, neater ones I used to accuse mentally of being "clothes horses" or "fashion plates."

Looking neat *as* I lose weight is part of my new dedication to my best self.

Let's try again: **I deserve to be thin.** And once more, with an echo: I DESERVE TO BE THIN. I deserve to be thin.

What can I do to send the FAT overcoat back to the second-hand shop?

(**Write your own specific program for change here.**) ____

_____

_____

_____

_____

_____

_____

_____

_____

_____

I wear my FAT as a clown suit

I am the jester, the joker, the funnyperson. Since FAT keeps me from being physically attractive, I become, instead, the one who clowns as a cover-up for hurts.

Long ago I discovered that people laughed at me for being FAT-and-funny. It was a negative sort of attention, to be sure. But it was attention. I have been clowning ever since. I am the one variety of heavyweight for whom the "fat people are jolly" phrase has some truth. For what the world sees is an affable, biggish person who plays at being the butt (the big butt) of others' jokes. Such sacrificing of self to the joke is the price I pay to be included in life's party.

I am not a nouveau-large. I have been heavy a long time. I have been wearing my FAT as a clown suit perhaps even since childhood. I may find it hard to step out of my clown role. How else will I win the applause I crave?

Conclusion: If I want to be a participant, not just a performer separated from my laughing public by a fence of footlights, I must doff my FAT clown suit, leave it in the circus ring where it belongs. I must recognize that I have real-person feelings and stop hiding them behind a loose laugh, a balloon suit, and a calliope shuffle.

Some specific ways to go about hanging up my clown suit: _____

_____

_____

_____

_____

_____

_____

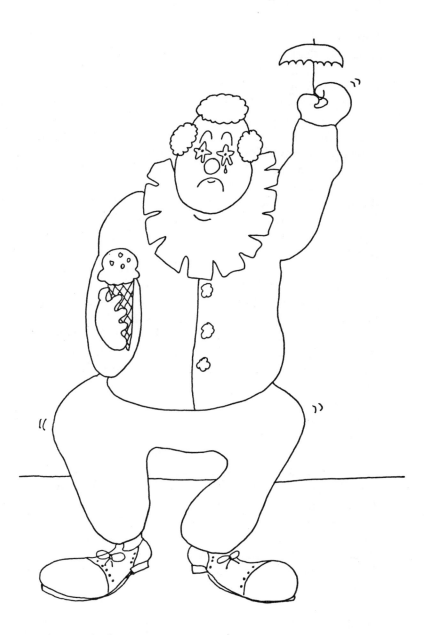

I clown as a cover-up for hurts

I wear my FAT as a weapon

I am a FAT rebel. I fairly bristle with FAT. Since fate has chosen to deal me out more than an ordinary dose of fatty tissue, I take out my heavy-hearted heaviness on everyone and everything.

I am the overscale teenager using my FAT to defy a parent, especially a normal-sized parent who has colossal expectations for me, who cares desperately about what I accomplish, how I look and what I wear, who regards my overweight as her/his own personal failure. With all the power of family-given authority, this parent tries to regulate my intake. Stocks the larder with visible diet foods. Keeps carrot sticks crisping in the fridge. Hides the sweets in the laundry room. Makes up elaborate weight charts. Offers rewards for pounds off — a peach-faced lovebird, a new bikini, fancy jeans, a season ticket to the hockey games, a trip to Disneyland.

Although I am dished up thinning foods at mealtime, between meals I escape to the nearest fast-food counter to take my place among the rest of the French-fried generation. Nothing helps. I have discovered that my FAT is one thing that no parent or other adult has any control over. Whoopee.

My FAT is a weapon. And I am miserable.

Although chronologically I may be well past the teen years, I may still be hung up in the FAT-is-a-weapon trap, the "getting back at" idea. (I may have trouble identifying whom or what I am getting back at.) Truth is, it is my own large self I am doing in. Who wants to be around a looming, hostile heavyweight?

I may be a wife getting back at a traveling husband. I may be a non-athletic brother getting back at a beautifully coordinated jock sister. I may be a grandmother getting back at her children and grandchildren because she feels neglected.

I need to recognize first of all that I am angry. I am FAT mad. I need to isolate those angers and deal with them in a new way — some other way that does not involve forking food into myself. Up to now, the madder I got, the FATter I got. And vice versa.

Sometimes a weight-losing fellowship can point out my angers and attitudes. Sometimes a professional therapist can help, especially one who has had a weight problem or who at least understands those who do. (Angry chubs have been known to become so infuriated at thin therapists that they have driven home by way of the bakery.)

If I recognize that I am using my own weight as a weapon, here is what I can do about it:

_____

_____

_____

_____

_____

_____

_____

_____

_____

_____

_____

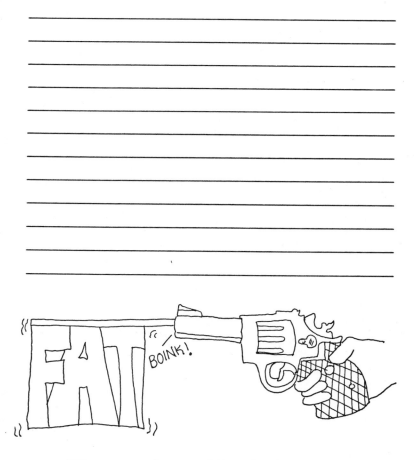

Whom or what am I "getting back at?"

I wear my FAT as a shroud

Am I shrugging off my right to a healthy life span?

Any near-blimp who continues on a dirigible course may come to as untimely an end as the Hindenburg itself. I know this. I have heard the "digging my grave with a spoon" line for years. But frankly, Gildenstern, it's hard to think of a teaspoonful of pudding in the same light as a shovelful of earth. A humming in my head keeps offering me false assurances: It can't happen to me. I keep right on overeating. Am I the FAT exception to columns of insurance statistics? Or am I, knowingly, destroying myself?

It is not pleasant to think that I am shrugging off my right to a healthy, reasonably lengthy life span, just by stuffing my face.

Do I really wear my FAT as a shroud? I am not consciously trying to do myself in. But like those other renowned compulsions, drinking too much alcohol and smoking, overeating is destructive. And I who overeat am self-destructive.

There is only one place to start — with my own attitude toward myself. I am a creature of God. I am a worthwhile human being. I deserve health, not destruction. I must have words with myself. One of the most important self-lectures of all is summed up in just three words:

I CHOOSE LIFE.

Humor Strategy

Play the simile game.

Start with yourself. I (in my oversize form) look like (choose one):

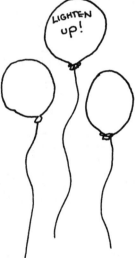

a mushroom upside down
three stacked-up Michelins
a divan
a double-dip cone
a spud
a bombay chest
a mallard
a banty rooster
a pear
a pair of pears . . .

    or think of something else.

Thin, I'm more like:

a celery stalk
a new moon
a ribbon

Use this same "is like a" game and apply it to pets, relationships, buildings, manners of speaking, whatever makes for an imaginative, just-for-laughter image. You'll find yourself smiling at the pictures you conjure up.

Things I can do better thin

Walk upstairs / Tie my shoes / Walk uphill / Pull on my socks / Make love / Scrub up muddy footprints / Play tennis / Play racquetball / Fix the roof / Play handball / Wash my hair frontwards over the basin / Scratch my back / Ride a bicycle uphill / Plant petunias / Pull dandelions / Pick potatoes / Give myself a pedicure / Pick burrs out of the dog / Water ski / Fit a pair of slacks / Wipe off the baseboards / Climb a ladder / Wrap a Band-Aid around a toe / Hang curtains / Go rock-climbing / Walk downtown / Look for a lost turtle / Pin up a hem / Catch a cab / Escape a mugger / Stay dry under an umbrella / Lay a carpet / Roll up a sleeping bag / Roll up *in* a sleeping bag / Roll up in a double sleeping bag / Hide Easter eggs / Become a mother / Become a father / Play jacks / Cook over a campfire / Shoot marbles / Play the accordion / Play the violin / Pick up spilled coffee beans / Chop wood / Swing a golf club / Wash a two-year-old in the tub / Wash a dog in the tub / Fit in the tub myself / Not spill on my tie / Shampoo the upholstery / Tend a fire / Climb in through the tailgate when I lock the the keys in the car / Find a four-leaf clover / Pick up shells / Pick up agates / Pick up a dime on the street / Run after a blowaway dollar / Change a tire / Hold a child on my lap / Hold a grown-up on my lap / Go curling / Fit in a telephone booth / Make a home run / Backpack / Put on a four-year-old's overshoes / Pull off a four-year-old's overshoes / Lay a patio / Climb a pasture fence / Jog / Get into an upper bunk / Board a train / Make a bed / Shovel snow / Change storm windows / Enjoy an intimate relationship / Look under the bed / Help a five-year-old roast a hot dog / Plant an apple tree / Thread a belt through belt-loops / Untree a cat / Pour a concrete floor / Disco dance / Ballet dance / Any kind of dance / Play volleyball / Sit at a counter / Run for a plane / Run for a bus / Run in a marathon / Just plain run / Have my appendix out / Have anything out surgically / Dine in a small cafe (with small tables and chairs) / Sit in a booth at a steak house / Get close to the kitchen sink / Get close to a photographer / Pose for a centerfold / Play quadruple solitaire on the floor / Find a girl friend / Find a boy friend / Clothe myself with half a yard of material / Do push-ups / Do chin-ups /

More?_____

_____

_____

_____

_____

_____

_____

_____

Things I can do better FAT:

Float

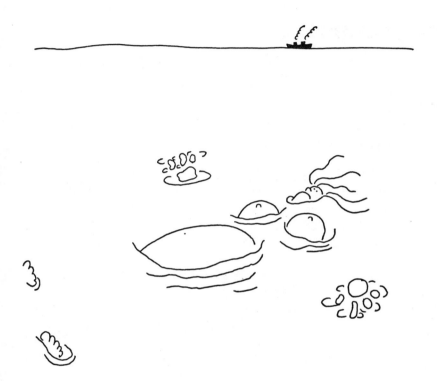

When you float, do you look like two volcanoes
and a large off-shore island?

Humor Strategy

Humor is an attitude — a way of opening up and seeing your situations and your surroundings. If you're not used to looking for what's funny around you, learn how, and laugh about it. (This doesn't mean to laugh at people's core beings — or appearances or characteristics they can't change. Healthy laughter is not unkind!)

Humor is part questioning.

Why is Miss Spandex with the maddeningly perfect body pausing so long in front of an overscale window mannequin in a shop for large sizes (an ironic reversal of the normal order of things!)

Why does the guy with the large, determined jaw choose a bulldog for a pet?

Why does the speech teacher look like her parrot?

Where do dwellers in cold climates *find* the garments that turn them into such silly bundles in the wintertime? Notice the man with three hats or the booted child in the padded snowsuit (she looks as if she's been blown up like a balloon with a tire pump). Notice the variety of muffler-wrapping techniques — from turban to holiday bow. On a below-zero day on a street, laugh at the people puffing steam like old locomotives and the wonderful variety of creatively warm, funny, human winter shapes! Quite a cloud you make too, especially if you're laughing!

Think of how funny you, yourself, must look, as you hide your oversized body in those comic, winter swaddles. By summer, you can change that oversize to normal size. Start now.

Learn to *see* what's funny. Laugh at yourself too. Laugh for the health of it.

A sink-side aside
in an appliance department

Said the salesman to Big Betty
As he pitched his wares, to wit:
Ma'am, you need a garbage disposer.
   She answered:
      I
         am
            it.

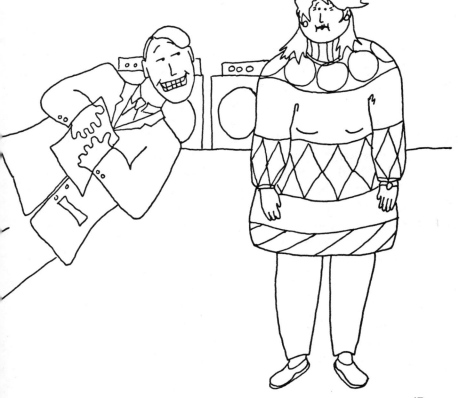

Classic types of overeaters

Are you here?

Am I a Sneakeater?

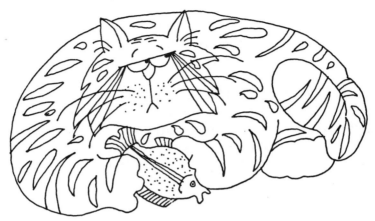

The Sneakeater is a light-fingered pickfridge.

Sneakeating is terribly important to this type of overeater. In fact, the sneaking may even be more important than the eating. Often Sneakeaters are reacting to the nagging of family and friends, especially long-term, predictable nagging. If every time you put food to mouth someone says, "You're not eating AGAIN!" or "All you DO is eat," that's enough to turn you into a Sneakeater.

In Sneakeaters, the most widely seen traits (of course, you don't SEE these traits — Sneakeaters won't let you) are greed and stealth. These food burglars come on little cat feet. They are masters at oh-so-silently opening cupboard and refrigerator doors. Their burgling expertise even extends to magnetized doors, the ones that grab at the last minute and suck themselves shut — with a bang.

You can spot Sneakeaters by their eagerness to carry out the supper dishes — all by themselves. Classic comment: "I'll do it. You don't need to help." Under the guise of serving others, they are serving themselves — the leftovers from every plate and platter.

Sneakeaters specialize in soft, silent foods: breads, preferably in plastic wrappers because paper bags crinkle, and noiseless spreads, spoonable sauces, quiet casseroles, mashed thises and thats, puddingish desserts. If temptation occasionally drives them to chew crunch food, they drown out the crunch by running the kitchen tap water. A Sneakeater in the kitchen has a common response to impatience from the dining area: "Just rinsing the dishes. Be there in a minute." This refrain is rendered hesitantly, between bites, but musically and with great good cheer.

Ordinarily Sneakeaters have sunny natures, unless somehow denied kitchen privileges.

Sneakeaters have well-developed hand-mouth coordination.

More than one Sneakeater in a household creates conflicts.

Some solutions for the Sneakeater:
1. Figure out how and when you sneakeat. (This is not easy, because you are probably so sneaky about food that you are fooling yourself, too.)
2. Vow to eat only at regular times and in the presence of others.
3. Sit down at a table when you eat.
4. Always eat from a plate and use a fork or a spoon — good discipline for the light-fingered pickfridge.
5. Wire each food cupboard with a buzzer set to jangle whenever the door is opened.
6. Equip yourself with winsome pets who wag or purr or snort so disarmingly while requesting leftovers that you cannot humanely deny them.
7. Let somebody else clear the lunch and supper tables.
8. Buy noisy food — celery, for instance. Sneakeaters resist noisy food. Even a potato chip sounds like a rifle crack to a sneakeater. But you'd better not take a chance on buying crackling chips, since a thwarted Sneakeater — give a little time and frustration — can be converted to a Cruncher, a defiant Food Rebel, who *likes* loud bites and doesn't care *who* hears them.

More help for the Sneakeater: _____

_____

_____

_____

_____

_____

_____

The Party-food Pass-up
Followed by the Stealthy at-home Snitch

"No thank you." We demur, and wave
Aside our good host's cooking.
Then later sneak our snacks at home
The minute no one's looking.

Am I a Nibbler?

The Nibbler delights in altering the symmetry of foodstuffs.

The Nibbler is a taster, a snitcher, a fingerlicker, who consistently prefers scraps, pieces, morsels, dibs and dabs to any sort of systematic mealtime eating.

I know I have Nibbler tendencies if:

I have a wild urge to pinch single pleats out of the fluted edge of the Great American Dessert. In fact, I have been known to divest this dessert of its entire top ruffle — one pleat at a time.

I leave bowling ball fingermarks in the tops of frosted you-know-whats.

I discover corners missing from food items in my refrigerator or bread box — ragged corners that smack of an infiltration of rodents. (Did *I* do that?)

Nibblers take subconscious delight in altering the symmetry of foodstuffs. They hark back to an earlier, less civilized age, in that they almost never use a fork or knife or spoon. Instead they count on the scoop effect of the single finger and the pincer properties of thumb and forefinger. Classic comment: a lip-smacking "Mmmmmmm," following a scoop-and-swallow.

A Nibbler eats lightly at meals — sometimes skips them altogether. ("I just don't seem to be very hungry.") A Nibbler complains a lot about how hard it is to lose weight. ("I don't understand it. I never eat that much.")

Nibblers can be dainty, since a couple of fingersful don't rake in much at a swipe. But calories, even in bits and licks, add up.

Nibblers could write a saga about their epic struggles against an overwhelming odd — namely a lifelong compulsion to nibble.

Question: What's a Wagnerian Nibbler's epic saga called?

Answer: ·pǝɥuǝƃunꞁǝꞁqqᴉN ∀

Suggestions for Nibblers:

1. Make a pact with yourself to eat only while sitting down at a set place at a table.
2. Eat only at specified meal times.
3. Until you break yourself of the thumb-and-forefinger pinching reflex, try eating only with a fork or spoon.
4. Design a good-sized ring to wear on your right forefinger (left forefinger if you're left-handed) and have it inscribed with STOP, FORBEAR, DESIST, or some other arresting command. Actually, any old ring would probably do the trick as a reminder.
5. Spend as little time as possible in the kitchen preparing food.
6. Those who have long regarded nibbling as a basic human need have trouble breaking the "must nibble" habit. If you feel driven to nibble, at least do so on low-calorie foods, like cut-up fresh vegetables. Try spearing an uncooked cauliflower or broccoli floweret with a fork. Perspire. Curse (mildly). Rise to new heights of small-muscle athletic endeavor. Don't give up. The secret cure for nibbling may lie in this empty (and you may be, too, by the time you accomplish it) challenge.

Your own program for change: _____

_____

_____

_____

Am I a Big Eater?

The Big Eater amazes people with his appetite.

The Big Eaters are usually men whose parents openly referred to them throughout their child- and teenhoods as Big Eaters.

"Eddie is a Big Eater, you know."

"I just don't know what I'm going to do to about that boy. I just can't seem to fill him up."

"I made a double batch, but the way that kid eats, they'll be gone in thirty seconds."

"He's a growing boy. And growing boys have incredible appetites."

All these statements are delivered with appropriate clucks and tsks and head shakes, frequently enough so that the kid does, indeed, think of himself as a Big Eater. He hears overtones of pride and amazement along with the clucks, and he begins to enjoy the distinction of having the biggest appetite in the family. It's fun to amaze people — a sure way of getting attention.

"Please pass the potatoes."

"Why Eddie, that's your FOURTH helping. Where do you put it all?"

And, where Eddie puts it becomes, to his delight, the general topic of conversation. Even if Eddie is not hungry, he feels compelled to overeat, just to maintain his Big Eater image.

Big Eaters were often wiry little boys who grew into strapping high school athletes. Then into college athletes. Then maybe into professional athletes.

"Where Eddie is putting it" becomes all too obvious when his level of activity drops, when he settles down as a sit-in-a-car salesman or a sit-at-a-desk executive. Little Eddie is now Big Ed. The wiry kid has been transformed into a paunchy, beefy adult, still living up to his lifelong notion of himself as the Big Eater.

Of course, the same kind of switchover to a sedentary lifestyle can affect the lanky girl athlete who ends up sitting at a desk eight hours a day.

"I can't understand it. I never had to think about weight before. I ate everything — EVERYTHING — just to gain weight."

The Big Eaters, who so happily astonished others with their extra-hearty appetites, wind up as astonished adults, dismayed at their own inflating shapes.

Were you a Big Eater as a child or a teenager? _____

Are you a Big Eater now? _____

Suggestions for Big Eaters:

1. Time to balance the caloric checkbook. This is one kind of classic overeater that may benefit from keeping track of calories. Somehow, the Big Eater has to regain the balance between energy used up and fuel taken in. When Big Eaters are no longer Big Spenders of calories, that's when the puff begins to gather.

2. If you have always exercised, don't stop now (except on medical advice). Find a substitute for football or track or hockey or whatever your sport was. If you can't afford a gym or a spa or a sports club, look for space to walk or run in. (There must be some free ground somewhere around.)

3. Make your three big squares three smaller squares. Obvious? Maybe, but it takes some doing. The guy in the habit of eating three suppertime rolls plus butter, for example — who buttered while he chattered — really has to concentrate on cutting back to one (or none).
4. Erase the Big Eater image, with all of its sub-images of the Big Athlete, the Tough Guy, the Kingpin, the magnanimous, the robust, the hale-and-hearty. You may be hearty, all right, if you keep up the Big Eater role, but you probably won't be hale. Instead, think of yourself, with pride, as one who "keeps in shape." Nothing is more visibly impressive than a big guy who has lost weight.

Any more ideas for Big Eaters? _____

_____

_____

_____

_____

_____

_____

_____

_____

_____

_____

Am I a Binge-eater?

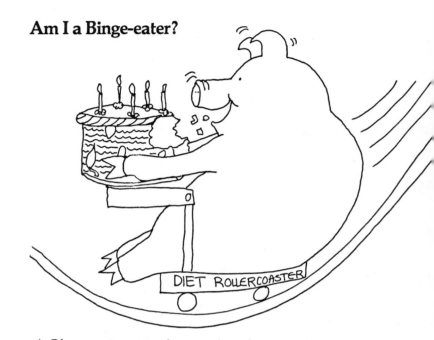

A Binge-eater needs to solve the puzzle of the guzzle.

Binge-eaters ride the seesaw. They are classic examples of the starve-and-stuff pattern. They are the least subtle of all overeaters, since it is hard not to notice someone who is indulging in food the way only a Binge-eater can.

Binge words: wolf, gobble, gorge, gluttonize, cram, grab, oink, guzzle, gormandize, stuff, glut, bolt, pig, splurge.

One who is engaging in any of the above has trouble maintaining a low profile.

Binge-eaters gain and lose the same old pounds, over and over and over again. They are likely to diet-to-eat-to-diet-to-eat-to-diet-to-eat-once-more. Their moods teeter in a direct ratio with their weight fluctuation. The pounds go down; the mood goes up. The pounds go up, the mood goes down. Discouragement and depression go along with bingeing.

Binge-eaters often profess to be sugarholics, too. Give them a teaspoon, and they'll take a cup. Several who binge admit to leading unscheduled lives, meals at funny hours, stretches with no food followed by splurges.

There are subcategories of Binge-eaters. The Weekender, for instance, who sticks stiffly by a diet program all week long and blows it from Friday night through Sunday. (The Weekender is also the always-on-Monday dieter.) The only way some Weekenders get ahead with a weight-losing plan is to lose more during the week than they gain back on the weekend.

The Night-eater is a daytime dieter whose motivation drops at nightfall.

The Late-afternoon Binge-eater topples off the diet at teatime, that horrendous, pre-supper children's hour (for some of us) which demands all of our resources at once. For the wife-mother or the wife-mother-worker, the hours of, roughly, 4 to 6 p.m., are the pits. We are mothers, wives, chefs, counselors, taxi-drivers, piano teachers, art consultants, math consultants, retrievers of lost sports equipment, menders of ripped jackets and scraped knees, dispensers of allowances, creative problem-solvers, noncreative problem-solvers, zookeepers — and Binge-eaters.

A binge-ing working man's day often peaks at the same time. He may come home and stuff on snackables. Or he may pub-stop and drink-and-eat a double load of calories.

A person who lives alone may discover that the lonely hours after work are binge times.

And the first thing a binge-ing teen does after school is to fly to the kitchen and fling open cupboards, refrigerator, breadbox, in quick succession, grabbing and gobbling all the way.

A big Binge-eater can remain binge-free for months at a time, then go on an overeating spree — a real lunatic binge — that may last a week or more. Needless to say, the weight from such an overfilling can be frightening.

What brings on a binge? We can guess, based on the experience of long-time Binge-eaters. Here are some answers from some who have tried to analyze their own reasons for binge-ing — in an attempt to solve the puzzle of the guzzle.

Overeaters Anonymous (in a sound piece of advice Borrowed from Alcoholics Anonymous) advises us not to get too Hungry, Angry, Lonely or Tired (HALT). Are any of these culprits behind your own splurges?

☐ Hunger (overweights seldom blame hunger for their overeating)
☐ Anger
☐ Loneliness
☐ Fatigue
☐ Boredom
☐ Anxiety
☐ Sadness
☐ Joy
☐ Guilt
☐ Relief
☐ Frustration
☐ Just because you're here and the food's here and oh, well . . .

Other _____

_____

_____

_____

_____

Suggestions for Binge-eaters:
1. Keep a tally of binges, when and where they happen, how you are feeling at the time, what you are doing. It may be just the analysis you need to change your

patterns. Almost all of us overeaters have some of the characteristics of the Binge-eater, at least part of the time. Understanding the circumstances of our binge-ing can help us overcome it.

2. If you are a Late-afternoon Binge-eater, eat a huge salad at 4:30 p.m.; avoid the pre-supper binge by first filling yourself up with rabbity greens.

3. If you are a Night-eater, get to bed — or to a gripping book — and ward off a late-evening food prowl. Decree: Make the kitchen out of bounds after supper.

4. If you are a Weekender, vary your weekend activi-ties. Don't hang around the house watching television with food in hand. Don't punctuate your dozens of Saturday house-mending chores with bouts of between-meals eating. Get involved with an activity — a sport or a task or a project — that holds your interest for a few hours. Leave the house, if need be, to escape the magnetism of the too-friendly fridge.

Any further ideas for Binge-eaters? Add them here: _____

_____

_____

_____

Inner rhymes from the binge-eater's manual

All of us
who binge —
we
well know:
It is time
to unhinge
the
elbow.

Am I a Grazer?

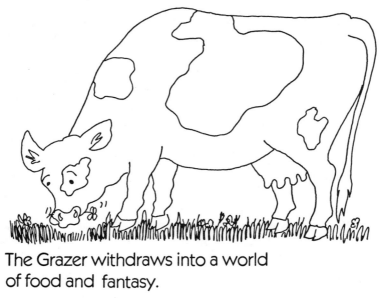

The Grazer withdraws into a world
of food and fantasy.

Grazers and Nibblers are alike in one way: They eat
almost all the time.

But whereas a Nibbler darts from food to food like a
hummingbird, consuming nervously and at high-speed, a
Grazer eats s-l-o-o-o-w-l-y. Grazers, like Big Eaters,
prefer to sit down and eat. A Big Eater, however, stations
himself at a table or kitchen counter, while you are more
apt to find a Grazer settled into a sofa or the Big Daddy
chair in the living room.

A Grazer is a combo eater, who engages in a constant
munch while watching television, doing homework, paying bills, listening to music or reading a book. A Grazer is
inclined to avoid family — even personal — responsibilities and withdraw into a world of food and fantasy.

Grazers are dreamy-eyed, placid, bovine in nature and
often lonely. Grazers are almost never in a hurry, even to
transport fork to face, but the forks seem to get there all
right — dependably, regularly, and often enough to keep
them at the overfill mark.

A Grazer usually plans ahead, taking time to prepare food, to mound a plate to its outermost rim with a "well-balanced" meal, before going at it. Therefore, a Grazer fares better nutritionally than a Cruncher (page 64), a Nibbler, a Sneakeater or a Binge-eater. The nutrition is okay; there is just too much of it.

Grazers like to do their own cooking. This makes sense because a Grazer would much rather eat alone than have anyone around making wonderstruck remarks about the size of helpings or the unbelievable number of apples or other goodies that have disappeared in a day. ("You mean you sat down and ate the *whole batch?*") He or she manages, through special scheduling, to partake of food at odd hours, thereby missing family meals — and family dishwashing.

Grazers are considered easy-going. They like their surroundings calm, lush and forever pleasant. For them, food is such a tranquilizer that they don't even seem to mind being barn-sized. But just shut a Grazer up in a stall, away from the fodder, and see what happens.

> One who grazes like a bovine
> Seems contented, although vast — sure.
> But a Grazer tends to grow mean
> When you take away the pasture.

Any of us who use food as a tranquilizer have Grazer tendencies. Suggestions for Grazers from former Grazers:
1. Rejoin the herd. Living in a fantasy world, withdrawn from people, is never as exciting as participating in the real one. This means developing new interests, new hobbies, new connections, new bridges to the outside. This is not easy. And it doesn't transform you overnight. But it is well worth the effort.
2. The first step toward recovering the reality of your own existence is to fill up your time. Don't allow yourself so much free, cooking-and-eating time.
3. Unhook the eating combos. Don't eat and watch television, or eat and read, or eat and write.

4. Eat at mealtimes, when others are present. A little self-honesty will tell you that your eating by yourself has less to do with a peculiar schedule than with hiding from other people's reactions to your overeating.

5. Join a diet group or fellowship. Lots of Grazers, along with other classic overeaters, have found their way to health through Overeaters Anonymous. OA's Program, based on the Twelve Steps developed by Alcoholics Anonymous, offers a Step-by-Step path to recovery from compulsive overeating. (And it's not a cowpath.)

If you are a Grazer, map your own route here for escaping from the barnyard: _____

_____

_____

_____

_____

_____

_____

_____

_____

_____

_____

_____

_____

_____

_____

_____

_____

_____

Chorus for a bucolic foodaholic

A romp
in the hay
beats
grazing —
any day.

Refrain for a Grazer

Refrain.

Am I a Cruncher?

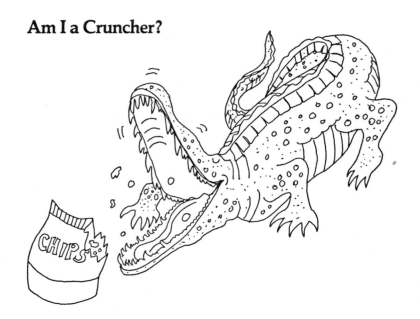

For the Cruncher, chomping is an act of defiance.

Nothing sneaky about this one. This noisiest of all overeaters is also the most resistant to change.

The Cruncher's loud chomping is an act of defiance. You can hear a Cruncher approaching from one flight up or a whole stoplight away — chewing raucously and crinkling noisy plastic or paper bags. Offspring of the original snap-crackle-pop cereal lovers, Crunchers are snackers on commercial non-mealtime extras — crackers, chips, tortillas and other big sellers with cute snack names.

When people around them cringe, or suggest that it's time to alter their eating habits, Crunchers turn warlike. In the mouths of these bellicose bellyfillers, a succession of chips becomes artillery, a box of crackers a barrage that is impossible to ignore. For a Cruncher can make a standard snack chip seem louder than it really is — in the wonderfully sound-engineered echo chambers of the mouth.

Crunchers' jaws crack a lot. They belch occasionally. Manners, even if they had learned a few somewhere along the line, have been overthrown by the rebel sounds of their own mastication.

They scatter trails of crumbs. (Pigeons follow them.) Their cars are carpeted in crumbs. Their beds prickle with them. A Cruncher crunching in a room can still all conversation, or necessitate cranking up the volume on the television.

Stress of any kind makes them crackle louder than ever. Let nobody tell a Cruncher what **not** to eat; it will have exactly the opposite effect. The classic attitude, although seldom expressed except in chews: "I'll eat what I like. And damn the consequences!"

In a household where a Cruncher lives, refrigerator doors are sprung. Cupboard door hinges work loose from sudden — loud — openings and closings.

Crunchers are angry people. They hide their pain under a semblance of "don't care," a macho image or a tough-bounce belligerence.

Check here if you think you have Cruncher tendencies often____ or now and then ____.

If so, what sorts of feelings bring out the Cruncher in you?

_____

_____

_____

What situations can turn you into a Cruncher, even temporarily?

_____

_____

_____

Note: According to one report, intake of crunch foods, such as packaged snacks, is up 85 per cent since 1935.

Suggestions for Crunchers:

1. It might help to know that you probably are an angry person, to accept your anger, identify it and express it. That's easy to say in one sentence, but it might require some serious work.

2. Find a group, like an Overeaters Anonymous or Emotions Anonymous meeting. You'll meet others there with feelings like yours. And the Twelve Steps (as developed by AA) will give you a systematic approach to your problems. The group shares, cares, and offers you the tools for change.

3. Make the switchover from chips to sugarless gum. You can crack it — depending on who's around to object — and not fatten yourself. Try other loud foods instead, like apples or celery or carrots or radishes, that are less caloric than crackersnacks

4. Clear the weight-producing crackle-foods out of your cupboards, your glove compartment, your desk drawer.

5. To start with, observe when and why you crunch, by writing down the times and how you feel when you do it.

6. Your goal is to restrict your intake to mealtimes, to cut out the pop-and-crunch between-meals snacking.

7. Like the Nibbler and the Grazer, you may benefit from eating only with utensils. Forget finger food. There is no way to fork a chip into your mouth.

Try to overcome your defiant eating by making the following changes:

_____

_____

_____

_____

_____

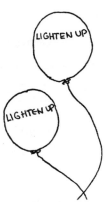

Humor Strategy

This comes from Dr. Dale L. Anderson, a simple way to get yourself to laugh and raise those endorphins:

At least once a day for, stand in front of a mirror (make that a full-length mirror) and laugh — not just quietly, but out loud. (You may want to be alone when you try this — unless you explain it first to those within earshot.)

Your laugh may start out sounding somewhat forced, but before long you'll find yourself genuinely laughing. You know how hard it is to keep from breaking up if others around you are folding over like omelettes with convulsive giggles or booming with uncontrollable mirth? You'll find that seeing and hearing *yourself* laugh will have the same effect!

When was the last time you were caught up in helpless laughter? Replace too-hearty eating with hearty laughter. It's very hard to laugh and eat at the same time.

Reshape your thinking:
Reshape your body

Misdefinition No. 1: Food is love.
Or, more specifically, sweet stuff is love. Baked things are love. Whatever is — no, whatever USED TO BE — my favorite edible is love. (And what made it my favorite edible? I linked it with love.)

We are trapped in a long literary and cultural tradition of the "food is love" idea, which began at our mothers' knees — or earlier. Here are some samples:

Patty cake, patty cake, baker's man . . .
Bake me a cake as fast as you can.
(Even in infancy I was ravenous — just couldn't wait!)
Pat it (tenderly) and roll it (lovingly)
And mark it with "B"
(Make that a double "B" — for Big Baby)
And put it in the oven for Baby and me.
(The suspense was terrible — so terrible, in fact, that I've been eating raw batter ever since. And wondering why a recipe that promises to feed eight emerges from the oven at MY house as barely enough to feed four and a half.)

Or:
". . . Visions of sugar plums danced in their heads."
(After all these years, are they still dancing in mine?)

Or some grown-up adaptations:
"Nothin' says lovin' like something from the oven."
(Have baked marvels replaced bundling?)
"If I'd known you were coming, I'd have baked a cake."
(For you? Or for me?)
"Sara Lee is love."
(Repeated o'er and o'er.)
Sara Lee is a mighty and successful food operation, but Sara Lee is not love.
"Armour makes it easy to say 'I love you' every day."
(There are other, perhaps better, facilitators of this kind of loving communication.)

What times in your life reinforced the "food is love" idea?

_____

_____

_____

_____

Redefinition:

Love is caring enough about my family and friends and my own going-on-thin self to avoid using food, especially FAT-making food, as a way of showing affection.

Some non-food ideas for indicating fondness for someone:
Gentle words show love.

A bunch of daffodils, bought on impulse from a sidewalk flower vendor, shows love.

A half-hour or so of undistracted listening shows love.

An appropriate little book shows love. Mark it at a place that reminds you especially of the person you care about.

Helping with a small (or large) task shows love.

Just taking time to remember occasions shared shows love.

A hug, a hand clasp, a smile shows love.

Think of other ways to prove that you care: _____

_____

_____

_____

_____

_____

_____

_____

Misdefinition No. 2: Food is a reward.

While "food is a reward" may not be a misdefinition for normal-sized folk, it certainly is for us FATS. This idea is a hard one to overcome because it is so creakingly ancient that it is ingrained in almost everything we do.

It goes back to a time when the reward of a long day's hunt was clubbing — and eating — your dinner. The reward of the back-bending work that goes into sowing and reaping crops has always been, of course, eating them. Even now, when food — at least for most of us — is relatively easy to come by, our first stop after the paycheck arrives is the supermarket. Food is the first reward for work.

Somewhere along the course of civilization, we added the concept that food is a reward for good behavior, for achievement in any field. There follows the modern institution of the Awards Banquet, where we hand out — along with chicken à la king — hockey letters, twenty-five-year watches, badges, diplomas, certificates and citations for everything from Motherhood of the Year to million-dollar life insurance sales.

Awards Dinners are so frequent that we have had to make room on our calendars (and in our bellies) for Awards Breakfast and Awards Luncheons, too. Since FATS often are doers, we must wage, along with our everyday FATfight, the never-ending Battle of the Banquets. How do you learn to live with these civilized bashes, these food-focused events? You eat the salads and drink the tomato juice and hope that the speeches end before you begin nibbling the edges of the creamed main dish or the dessert tarts.

As doers and achievers, many of us are grown-up Good Girls and Good Boys who consistently have been rewarded since childhood with food — usually gooey, sugary food. "If you're good, I'll give you some hmmmm-hmmmm." Are we doing the same thing to our own children?

How about the early input from nursery literature?

The bad little kittens' cat mother said:

"What? Found your mittens, you good little kittens?

Then you shall have some pie."

Little Tommy Tucker was rewarded for singing with a supper of white bread and butter.

Little Jack Horner in his corner, as he ate his Christmas pie, "put in his thumb and pulled out a plum and said, 'What a good boy am I!' "

Good kids get good goodies to eat. Everybody from Mother Goose on up says so.

Often a food reward bears absolutely no relation to what is being rewarded. It may be totally inappropriate, just an automatic response.

"You say you won the week's Most Pounds Off award at the spa? That calls for your favorite desert!" WRONG!

"Nancy was chosen Miss Health at college. I think I'll send her a cake with 'Congrats, Miss Health' on it." Miss Health, if she is true to her title, probably won't eat it, but her dorm chums will.

The most common manifestation of food as a reward is the grand old tradition of the cake. You get a high-rise model for getting married. Simpler versions mark every kind of human milestone or accomplishment: "flying up" from Brownie to Girl Scout, recovering from a cold, graduating (from anyplace), getting admitted (to anyplace from stewardess school to the state bar), bringing home a new baby, signing up a new client, climbing a mountain, winning a race, selling a lot of goods, getting your cast cut off, earning an A+, having a Bar Mitzvah, being confirmed, moving out, moving in, switching careers, being promoted, growing the state's biggest squash — or simply living through another year.

Check here if you have heard these food-as-a-reward — or food-as-a-bribe — statements directed to you. Double check any that you may have not only heard, but also said:

☐ "Eat your spinach (brussels sprouts, carrots, rutabagas), and you can have some dessert."

- ☐ Or the negative version: "If you *don't* eat your spinach (etcetera), you *won't* get any dessert."
- ☐ When you finish your homework, I have a treat for you." (An incredible edible of some kind.)
- ☐ "Well, I'm certainly not cooking supper until you're through mowing the lawn!"
- ☐ "You kids have worked so hard painting the place that you deserve to go out somewhere and have a really good meal."
- ☐ "If the team wins this game, we'll stop at Wafflechompers on our way back to school." (Understood: If we lose, we don't get our syrup-drenched reward.)

Add here any situations or remarks you remember that reinforced the idea of food as a reward:

_____

_____

_____

_____

_____

_____

_____

Let's vary the theme. If rewards must be food, substitute a big bowl of fruit or homegrown vegetables for baked and frosted things. Instead of dribbling the sentiments in icing script, plant a flag with the same message in an apple or a grapefruit or a royal-red cabbage. Or drape a printed ribbon around a beautiful eggplant.

Whenever you need a happy-anything noncake, experiment. Try a minimally caloric Frosted Jiggle of layered gelatin made with diet pop or fruit juice. A thick frosting of egg whites beaten stiff with sugar substitute, flavoring and cream of tartar will anchor birthday candles. This won't win a bake-off prize, but it will elicit an initial "Gee, it's a cake!" reaction from celebraters. Such Jiggles may help us get rid of our own.

Or consider nonfood rewards. Choosing the just-right reward for a special accomplishment becomes a marvelous challenge. If you are a parent, start thinking NOW about nonfood rewards for your children. Maybe you can help them steer clear of the roly-poly doldrums in their teen years.

Add your own rewards ideas to this brief list:
    a miniature painting
    a piece of sculpture
    a hand-thrown pot
    a book
    a hilarious pair of socks
    an engraved medallion or charm
    a handmade trophy
    a clock
    a scrolly certificate
    a hand-stitched wall banner
    a potted tree
    an evening of music or theater
    tickets to a game
    a poster signed by all concerned
    a scarf or tie embroidered with names of all concerned
    anything permanent engraved with a personal message

_____

_____

_____

_____

_____

_____

_____

Q What would you call an overweight swinger from the Twenties?

A. *A flabber*

Misdefinition No. 3: Food is fun.

Just try to get around this one: Food is fun — a picnic in a park, a supper by candlelight, a sweet lunchtime escape from a business day, a swoop through a drive-in, a surprise in an ethnic restaurant, a gathering of good friends at supper, a whispered-over dinner for two.

No party worth its parsley is minus food. Who can invite anyone anywhere without offering a nibblet with a drink or some new concoction on a buffet table? From "Come on over for supper" to "Mr. and Mrs. Gadding Hailfellow request the pleasure of your company," it is well understood that food is the necessary element. Food means festivity, and festivity means fun.

Try some alternatives. Invite friends over for:
- A kite fly
- A haying party
- A walk through a park
- An outdoor musicale
- A tea-tasting party
- Cross-country skiing
- Old movies
- A vegetable-garden planting party (great for city folk — give them each a corner of the plot, then invite them back for the harvest)

Other ideas for entertaining: _____

_____

_____

_____

_____

_____

_____

_____

_____

_____

Misdefinition No. 4: Food is a responsibility.

"It's a sin to waste food."

While we were drumming our little curly-handled spoons on our high-chair trays, our elders were drumming this principle into our heads. We have felt guilty ever since about being FAT in a hungry world. As we listened to those sad-and-true tales about starving children, we were shaping ourselves into anything but. With a happy sense of duty, we ate our way to the bottom of the bowl to uncover the picture of the three little pigs. Only with the dawning of adulthood, did we pause to ponder the question: Just how did overfeeding our own faces help solve the terrible problems of world hunger?

For some of us who were children during the 1930s Depression, food meant survival. Dust storms coated our window sills with reddish silt. Boxcar riders from the nearby freight yards and "hobo jungles" knocked at our doors asking for handouts. We were frightened by the look of hunger on those gaunt faces. Even though we were the lucky ones who had enough to eat, we were aware that the greatest gift we could give another human being was food. A drumstick and a piece of pie offered on the back steps outside the kitchen was as much a marvel as a pirate's chest loaded with glinting pieces of eight.

Are we still thinking of every bite as a treasure?

Are those early biddings and urgings to eat-it-all-up because somebody else is hungry still whispering to me as I, ensconced in my favorite restaurant, eat every shred of lettuce dished up to me, every last one of the prepackaged crackers, every crust and crumb in the bread basket?

Are we grown-up members of the World War II Clean Plate Club? During those years of total mobilization, it was not only a horror to waste food, it was also unpatriotic. Have we been responsibly polishing our plates with our forks since then? Are we caught between two sins: the sin of wasting food and one of the seven deadlies — gluttony?

To unlatch our storehouse of guilt — and guilt gets in

the way of thinning — here's a thought: Keep track of how much money you save in a month out of the food budget when you are dieting. You will save money. Although the food you are buying may be more nutritious and more expensive, you are buying a lot less of it. Mail a check for the difference between your weight-watching food budget and your eat-everything-you-can-lay-your-hands-on budget to one of these organizations (or another of your own choosing), which are working to end hunger in the world.

World Vision International
P.O. Box O, Pasadena, California 91109
(Specify to "help feed the hungry.")

The Hunger Project
2015 Steiner Street
San Francisco, California 94115

Of course, it is immoral to waste food (and restaurants are the worst wasters). But putting it in our already overloaded, unfit bodies is no solution.

FAT and feelings

When others have fits, we have FATS

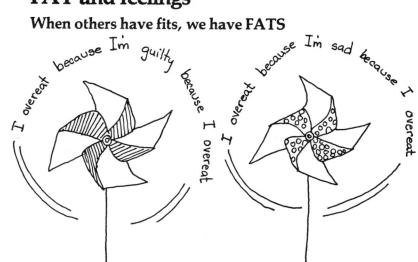

I overeat because I'm guilty because I overeat

I overeat because I'm sad because I overeat

FAT and feelings mingle in so many ways that we overweights sometimes feel like the pins in a succession of pinwheels, all spinning and circling in an endless whir and getting nowhere.

We overeat because we are angry because we overeat.

We overeat because we are sad because we overeat.

We overeat and are overcome with guilt. Then we overeat *because* we are overcome with guilt from overeating. And on and on to a FAT end.

Oh-so-often overeating is our way of handling anxieties and stress. Others break out in tremors, cold sweats and ulcers. We break out in FAT. When others have fits, we have FATS.

A lot of us are firm (plenty firm) believers in self-control, in not allowing our feelings to surface and show. If we are lifelong heavies, we doubtless learned that kind of control early while coping with the taunts of thin children. It was bad enough to be a fatso without being a crybaby, too. That would have given our taunters ammunition for a double-barreled assault. Some of us took the classic "big girls (big boys) don't cry" remark literally. To be a "big girl" or a "big boy" meant to please our elders by being a large-sized stoic. Are we still toting those old tags around with us in our adulthood?

Sometimes we feel that because we are FAT we are not *allowed* to have the usual rainbow of emotions — from anger to fear to shame to joy to sadness to love. We are intended to be bystanders. We are so big and mighty that any display of emotional fireworks seems inapproriate and embarrassing.

Several of us OWs carry this control further still and try to control other people. We are often manipulators. We rule our roosts quietly, but we control them neverthe-less, sometimes by a seeming *lack* of control. An infor-mal poll of several overweights in one diet fellowship brought forth the admission from exactly half of them that they did, indeed, feel that they were "controllers," not only of their own subdued emotions, but of others' lives. What could be more depressing for me, the control-ler, than a situation (my own overweight) that has gotten out of hand, one in which I feel helpless? It's enough to drive me to a self-defeating journey to the Gorge of the FATfolk.

A dimensional dirge

When you call attention
With condescension
To the extra size of my thickness through,
Such casual mention
Of my third dimension
Makes me wish I had only two.

A dump for old FAThurts

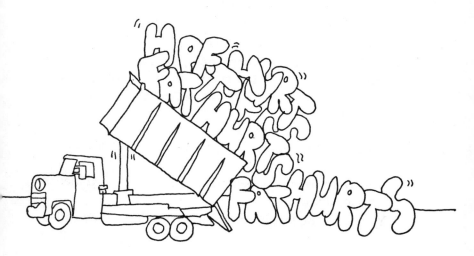

Taunts, jibes, barbs, teases from thin peers, whatever their age, tend to ring in FAT ears forever. These wounds are blocks in the way of our thin renewal. They are always with us, as part of our self-portraits, pulling us down in our own estimations, keeping us — out of sheer discouragement — from making the best of ourselves.

Dig up those old FAThurts. You will be astounded at how many wounding phrases can be resurrected, intact, complete with tone and inflection. Gentle words melt in the memory after a time. (Try to remember the nice things people have said about you, and see how hard it is to dredge them up.) But harsh words seem to petrify and become artifacts, preserved for all time in our personal history museums. Gather them from their ancient showcases. Dump them out — here. And forget them. It's museum-cleaning time.

Are any of these FAThurts — or similar ones — still with you? Check those you can relate to. Then add your own.

If you were an apple-shaped child:

☐ Recess at school — gym class, too — became your own private, everyday hell.

☐ You were always the last one picked when they chose up sides for any kind of game.

☐ You got caught in jump ropes, because gravity was too much for you. And every time you did, the other kids hawhawed or made up jump-rope jingles about you.

☐ You "missed" so often at hopscotch, because you were big and off-balance, that you gave up and sat on the curb.

☐ You were four laps behind the rest in the President's Physical Fitness sprints.

☐ You were the last holdout on a tricycle — they called you Trikie Mikie — because it wasn't easy to learn to keep your bulk from toppling a two-wheeler.

☐ In school plays, you were always type-cast as Jack Sprat's wife, Peter's pumpkin, somebody's comfy grandmother, a tree, a fat shoemaker, a clown, or the moon.

Other: _____

☐ The teachers always counted on you for behind-the-scrim tableau scenes because you could sit so still. (Young FATS are not wigglers.)

☐ You were the only FAT fairy (elf) in the second grade play. You didn't fit your costume, so they made you into a mushroom instead.

☐ Other kids called you names:

Two-ton	Lardy
Semi	Blubberbutt
Moby	Fatso
Dumbo	Fatty Arbuckle
Moonface	(if you're over 50)

Fatty-fatty-two-by-four
   Can't-get-through-the-kitchen-door
Blimp
Hippo
Jumbo
Leadbottom
Other labels meaning large:

_____

_____

_____

_____

Check one:

☐ You bore these slings and arrows in stunned silence.

☐ You retaliated in kind, calling your thin taunters: skinny minnies, sticks, scrawnies, boneys, bag o' boneses, scarecrows, broomsticks, pipe cleaners. But you couldn't muster much conviction. In fact, you would have given anything — anything but your sweets and snacks — to be a pipe cleaner yourself.

Q: What did you call your sister when she told your mother that you sneaked off to the soda fountain and ate a frozen-island-in-a-tub with a double dip of glop on it?

A: _A FAT Telltale_

If you were — oh, the humiliation of it all! — a tubby teen:

☐ Well, first of all they all _called_ you a tubby teen — and you shrank (in every way except literally) from the label.

☐ You felt left out of things, because you overheard someone say, "Of course (your name here) is too FAT to go with us" — on a hike, on a hayride, waterskiing, cross-country skiing, rock-climbing, potato-picking, swimming or any other activity less suitable for FAT kids than thin ones.

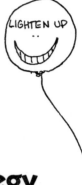

Humor Strategy

Look back in laughter. Today's disasters will all have their lighter moments, when viewed in retrospect. Pick up on the inherent humor in a situation and remember it — someday you'll laugh.

As for today — remember past disasters or times of chaos and laugh about *them* now.

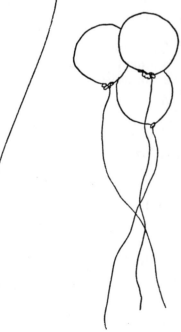

Recall any such instance? _____

_____

☐ On so many Saturdays the girl next door asked you the same terrible question, "Are you going to the dance tonight?" (Make it a sock hop or a disco, depending upon the particular decade your teenhood spanned.) And you had the same mortifying answer. "No, are you?" Why did she ask? She knew you would be stuck at home as usual (listening to "Your Hit Parade" on the radio, or watching "Emergency" or "Horror Incorporated" or "Saturday Night Live" — again depending on the era).

☐ You were the butt of FAT jokes. (The elephant joke fad was especially hard on heavy teens.)

☐ You had a few friends, but you weren't anybody's sweetheart.

☐ You had one very glamorous or handsome, very popular friend. But you suspected all along that she (he) kept you around for contrast, as a sort of pilot fish.

☐ When everybody else wore jeans, they teased you about wearing stretch pants.

☐ Your mother said, like a stuck-in-a-groove record, "You're not going to eat THAT, are you? Don't you have any will power?" (Of course, you went ahead and ate it.)

☐ The gym teacher said, eyeing you critically, "I think it's time we (editorial "we") went on a diet."

☐ And then there was the crushing day when you discovered that your mother (father) wore a whole size smaller than you did.

There were other, excruciating remarks or situations, perhaps too humiliating to recall. But try to remember them. Find them. Then, in one final heave-ho, toss them out.

How about as an adult — do any of these remarks sound familiar?

- ☐ "You look like a Rubens." (A 16th-17th century Flemish painter who liked his women pink and huge.) From your husband — who does not.

- ☐ "You look like a Lachaise" (Worse yet, referring to a sculptor whose women were positively monumental.) Also from the male body-critic in your life.

- ☐ "I would have thought you'd have more pride than to let yourself get so FAT." From a spouse who can eat everything in sight and never worry about pride or lack of it.

- ☐ "Are you still FAT?" From somebody you knew you as a plump adolescent and hasn't seen you since.

- ☐ "If you were thinner, I'd marry you." From the girl (boy) who has been your lifelong friend and sometime lover.

- ☐ "Your mom (dad) is a blimp." From your child's constant playmate. Reported by your child.

- ☐ "You have a big seat." Matter-of-fact statement from teenager hanging out car window and passing you on your bicycle. (Translate into teen-ese.)

- ☐ "You're F-A-A-A-T!" Toddler at the beach.

- ☐ "And who are you? I didn't catch the name . . . " A former classmate who draws a blank at the sight of you in an airport.

- ☐ "WHEN are you going to do something about your weight?" (Spouse, parent, well-meaning friend, co-worker, boss, doctor, coach, offspring, grand-offspring.)

What else hurts? _____

_____

_____

_____

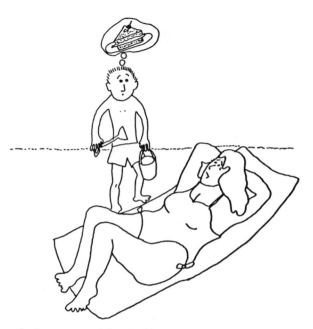

Your father says I look like a Rubens.

Moments of derision can be moments of decision

Some of the old FAThurts can be recycled into constructive energies — if I have decided, once and for all, to stop feeling sorry for myself as a pin cushion for needling remarks. I will turn my emotional bruises into angers. Angers at my FAT (not at the insensitive ones who did the needling).

The good old, "I'll show THEM," burn can be enough to spark beginning a new diet-exercise program. But it takes more than smoldering to keep me on it. It takes positive thoughts — convincing myself that "I am doing this for ME." Not for my husband, who would like a wife he can be proud of — with new people as well as with those who already accept me as an okay, though large, person. Not for my wife, who fusses about my health. Not for the kids. Not for the doctor. Not for the insurance agent. FOR ME, MYSELF.

Am I padding my body with a Guilt Quilt?

Woe to us who make a habit of feeling guilty, for we are headed for a puffed-up future self unless we stop stuffing our personal Guilt Quilts!

A little guilt is tolerable — just enough to keep us ethically upright and morally comfortable. But we, the superguilty and superpadded, spend too many of our thoughtful moments kicking ourselves (a neat trick for a FATty) for what we *should have* done.

We add to our pillowy exteriors with Guilt Quilts. Every offspring's tear or disappointed, "Aw, gee," every parent's reprimand, every colleague's impatience, every spouse's sigh of irritation, every whine, every meow — even if I am not the immediate cause — so stifles me with guilt that I turn to food. A drooping philodendron (dumb dingdong me! I forgot to water the plants!) has been known to set off an all-day guilt binge.

Each one of these "should have's" is worth one or more puffy square(s) on my Guilt Quilt: (And if a square is equal to a pound . . .?)

☐ I *should have* picked up Buzzy after basketball practice instead of letting him walk home in a blizzard. (Flu kept him off the team.) One square.

☐ I *should have* looked for the cat that night he disappeared, instead of racing off to my bowling league. (The kids were heartbroken.) Two squares.

☐ I *should have* coached that trainee before he walked in to confront the manager. (He's not working here anymore.) One square.

☐ I *should have* handed the Heart Fund envelope to my neighbor instead of sticking it in her door. (Where is it now?) One square.

☐ I *should have* cooked more interesting meals for my family; then maybe they would have spent more time at home. (Now it's too late.) Three squares.

☐ I *should have* held out for more money, trained myself for a better job, stuck with the company, left the company, planned for our retirement, invested more shrewdly. (Now we're strapped.) Four squares — or more.

☐ I *should have* washed the baby's head more often. (She's showing signs — how embarrassing! — of cradle cap.) Two squares.

☐ I *should have* offered to drive Aunt Emily to the eye doctor the day she fell at the bus stop. (She's in a cast.) Two squares.

☐ I *should have* known the neighbor child was in trouble and warned the parents before the police came. (The police came.) Three squares.

☐ I *should have* volunteered to babysit for my grandchild, so that his mother could go to law school. (But it has taken me sixteen long years to learn to live without animal crackers. I just can't restock my cupboards with high binge-potential baby snacks.) Five squares.

☐ I *should have* asked the new minister (new neighbor, new teacher) over for dinner (out for lunch). One square for each "new" person ignored.

☐ I *should have* given more time to my children (spouse, parents, old minister, old teacher). One square for each "old" person slighted.

☐ I *should have* written my sister. One square.

☐ I *should have* written my mother. One square.

☐ I *should have* continued my education. Three squares.

☐ I *should have* put the education I had to better use. Three squares.

☐ I *should have* sewed up that ski jacket, fixed the kitchen screen, cleaned my desk, mowed the lawn, yanked the weeds — or done any other humdrum task that I put off doing until someone else had to do it. One square each.

☐ I *should have* been a better wife, husband, mother,

father, boss, worker, student, lover, whatever. Two squares each.

☐ And probably the biggest "should have" of all: I *should have* checked my overeating long ago, before I put on all this extra weight. Make this ten squares. Make it a center design in my personal Guilt Quilt.

Add your own list of "should have's" here. The more pounds you have added over the years, the more squares you'll need — and the bigger and puffier your quilt will be:

I should have   I should have

_____ _____

_____ _____

_____ _____

I should have   I should have

_____ _____

_____ _____

_____ _____

I should have   I should have

_____ _____

_____ _____

_____ _____

I should have   I should have

_____ _____

_____ _____

_____ _____

Once I have identified and labeled the squares in my Guilt Quilt, I will try to forget them. Lingering guilt is

I should have...

waxed the car

called my Aunt on her birthday*

Studied harder

paid my bills

said I was sorry

patted the dog

smiled

been more understanding

stuck to my diet

been on time for the meeting

called back when I said I would

waved

tipped the waitress even though the service was lousy

shingled the roof

carved a national monument on my day off

been a better person

Guilt Quilt

unproductive — and it does not, in the long run, help anyone lose weight. If I come upon any of these "should have's" that are still feathering my quilt, and if it is possible to make amends, I will do so. Do them and erase them. If I can't get out and take care of these old "should have's," at least I can share my feelings about them. I'll tell somebody — preferably another OW, who will understand. If this is impossible, I will write it as a diary entry. Maybe that will help take the guilt-stuffing out of my quilt.

Some pound-sparing thoughts: I only feel as guilty as I allow myself to feel. Could it possibly be that I *like* to feel guilty?

Grown-up "good girls" and "good boys" are particularly skillful at stitching together Guilt Quilts. If I have a FATtish family, maybe we all are involved in a nonstop, floating guilt-quilting bee.

I will match up the times I oversnack and overstuff with my feelings of guilt. I may be surprised at how guilt and eating can conspire together for my downfall.

FAT irony

If I don't eat much of it,
I am more likely to be called it.

Honey / sugar / lambchop / muffin / sweet stuff /
other sugar-frosted terms of endearment.

From padded FAT to unprotected thin

When we begin to trim down somewhat, the extent of our former non-feeling becomes apparent. We are surprised, after peeling off some of the padding and cutting down on our tranquilizer (food), at the emotional explosions that pop out of our thinner selves. Actually, we are more than surprised; we are stunned and blinking to hear our own voices professing anger, ("but I *never* get mad at anything") or admitting to others that we care about them.

We have been such people-pleasers, such smoothers of the waters, such avoiders of strife that we have to learn to deal with this new assertiveness, this new respect of ours for our own emotions.

Some comparisons illustrate what happens when we go from a padded FAT to an unprotected thin. The risks are huge (but better an enormous risk than an enormous body).

FAT

Sad, I eat, of course. There is no way to escape sadness, but I have spooned into myself more than an ordinary dose of it by being overweight. Overweight **is** sadness. So are other things, like death, parting, divorce, loss, a dream unrealized, a potential unfulfilled.

I am weighed down, not only by the cares of the world, but by my own pounds. But I certainly would never let on about how sad I am. That would admit my weakness. A big person is supposed to be strong.

Thin

Sad, I will realize that there is nothing wrong with being sad. If I feel sad. I will recognize my sadness as a fact. It is not shameful to show sadness. As a child, if I was sad, I was hushed up with food. I will no longer "treat" sadness with food. I'll allow myself to feel the pain.

FAT

Angry, I eat. I am, after all, the good guy (girl) who never gets angry, the one who is always smoothing others' ruffled feathers. Never mind my own. I'm not sure I even know what real anger feels like anymore . . .

Guilty, I eat — and eat and eat. Much of my guilt has to do with being a compulsive overeater and an overweight person. I live my life in a perpetual state of guilt — over what I have *not* done for other people, or what I *have* done to myself. The guiltier I feel, the more I eat. And I set in motion the most pernicious pinwheel of all!

Thin

Angry, I will recognize my own anger. It's there, all right, if I will just let myself feel it. I know, from the patterns in my past, that I cannot allow that anger to seethe inside without overeating. I will try to say, "I am angry," and explain why. If expressing my anger is not practical (what if I lose my job for blowing up at the boss?), I'll try to find other ways to handle it. I'll run it off, or rush around a tennis court, play Black Mountain Rag on my banjo or pour a concrete garage floor or scrub a wall.

Guilty, I'll look at my guilt and see it for what it is — a stumbling block. As I start to lose weight, some of this terrible guilt begins to leave me. I am trying, and I am losing.

As for those undone "should have's" (see the Guilt Quilt), I'll either stop stewing and *do* them or I'll make it clear why I choose not to.

FAT

Depressed, I eat because I feel so helpless in my sadness that there seems to be no way out of this mess. Who cares if I'm FAT? Even I don't care what happens to me. I am a round robot, just going through the motions of existing.

Hurt, I eat, and nobody knows how I really feel. It is embarrassing for a heavy person to act hurt.

Joyful, yes, even happy, I eat. Food is what celebration is all about, isn't it? And how can I pass up all those good celebration foods? Other people would think I didn't care about their celebrations if I didn't eat. And I certainly don't want to hurt anyone's feelings.

Bored, I eat. Life is dull because I am a dull, heavy person. As long as I am carrying around a prison of extra weight, I am limited in the things I can do.

Thin

Depressed? Helpless? I will try to make the necessary choices to change some of the things I can. My weight, for instance. I will learn about where to go for help — spiritual or professional or both. I will admit that I need friends, that a sadness shared is a sadness soothed.

Hurt, I will acknowledge my hurt. If that hurt is building barricades in a relationship, I will talk about it — even put aside pride and bring up my feelings to the person(s) involved.

Joyful, Happy, I will find other, nonfood ways to celebrate my joy. Just being thin is a celebration of joy.

Bored, I will recognize — perhaps all in a flash — that I don't *need* to be bored anymore. The world is opening up for me, and I see choices — wonderful

FAT

Thin

choices. Things to do. People to meet. A new freedom to test — my freedom from FAT.

Afraid, I eat. Anxious, I eat. Scared to death, I eat. Others may pace, wring their hands, fret in a million nervous ways. But I eat. Food is my solace, my friend, my escape. It keeps me from facing up to frightening situations — not the least of which is my own overweight.

Afraid, I will admit it. Anxious, I will make an effort to find other ways to deal with the kind of stress that used to set me to nibbling. Prayer? A walk? A run? A dance? A swim? Biofeedback? Meditation? Any of several effective methods of self-psyching. Anything but eating.

In love, I hide and eat. Since any relationship is likely to be a one-sided infatuation, there is no point in letting the object of the infatuation know about it. I have been rejected too many times. Much better that I don't invest too much of myself in a hopeless romantic cause. (And there is so much of me to invest!) I'll just eat instead.

In love, my chances are as good as anybody's, not just because I am thinner and more appealing to others than I used to be as a bubble-shape, but because I have a new self-confidence, a new joy that makes me more interesting to be around. I like myself. Why shouldn't someone else like me?

Things are looking up as the weight goes down. I feel a whole range of emotions. Oh, yes, I feel them all right. But they are simpler, somehow, less confused. I can look at them more honestly, now that I am heading in a thin direction. I have discovered that I don't have to be caught in the middle of those crazy pinwheels. I can stop their spinning, just by making the decision to change the shape I'm in.

Humor Strategy

When you hear laughter, you laugh. So one of the most sure-to-spark-laughter strategies is simply to be around laughter.

Any child under three who is really laughing is guaranteed to infect you with laughter.

A comedy club with a clever comic artist may catch you up in waves of audience laughter.

Even laughter captured and recorded in a "laughing toy" can set you off.

Or go outside, to a place with lively nature sounds, and listen. A brook doesn't babble; it laughs. Those birds aren't singing; they're laughing!

Visualize people you love laughing.

Be part of that natural laughter. Laugh along. Picture yourself as a light-hearted — and lighter — person, laughing.

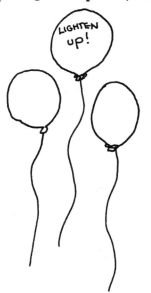

Phase out the FAT phrase, or in other words . . .

Food words are staples in our language — even when they don't actually apply to food. Food images pepper our conversations. They sweeten our phrases of endearment. They spice up our business dealings. They are the frosting on the cake of our communication.

If we are trying to watch our food intake, these can be tough to swallow. Let's lay them on the table. Following each food word of phrase or figure of speech is a blank. Just to preserve ourselves from unwanted cues to eat, how about trying to think of another way to say the same thing in nongastronomical terms, less tasty perhaps, but safer.

Example:

George is bringing home the bacon. _George has a good job_

Henry knows his onions. _____

She knows what side her bread is buttered on. _____

A fine kettle of fish (somewhat archaic). _____

Are you putting all your eggs in one basket? _____

What's that got to do with the price of beans? _____

She's chicken. _____

She's a chick. _____

Just like taking candy from a baby. _____

It's the spice of life. (What is?) _____

Everybody wants a piece of the pie. _____

Phyllis is flat as a pancake. _____

This fog is thicker than pea soup. _____

Annie's in a real stew. _____

Pretty please with sugar on it. _____

Alice has a cookie in the oven. _____

Who's a cornball? _____

Sam has cauliflower ears. _____

She's the cream in his coffee. _____

He's a real marshmallow. _____

Who's a milktoast? _____

You might try to butter him up. _____

He's not worth his salt. _____

Cool as a cucumber. _____

Move your buns. _____

That's a hot potato. _____

Nuttier than a fruitcake. _____

One rotten apple spoils the barrel. _____

Easy as pie. _____

She knows how to cut the mustard. _____

It's a real rhubarb. _____

Milk it for all it's worth. _____

Offer him a carrot. _____

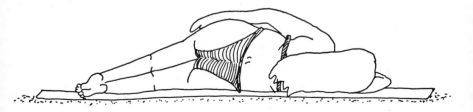

Fat cells by the sea shore

Heather has a peaches and cream complexion. ___ ___ . ___ ___

Her new job is a real plum. _____

Hot dog! _____

You turkey! _____

Too many cooks spoil the broth. _____

Mon petit chou. _____

He has a legitimate beef. _____

We need to beef it up. _____

He's a shrimp. _____

A hard nut to crack. _____

It ain't peanuts. _____

I'm in a pickle. _____

I can't see *that* for sour apples. _____

It's a case of sour grapes. _____

Albert is in the sauce. _____

That's a lotta lettuce. _____

He got me right in the chops. _____

Ronald is a ham. _____

We can put on weight just by thinking these food-centered thoughts — and letting them trigger our appetites. Most of us OWs would be better off putting all of these food images on the back burner.

More food imagery that needs revising: _____

_____

_____

_____

_____

_____

The geographical dilemma of where to put my belt — high on the hips, low on the hips, or someplace north of both

I think
I'd better
deflate or
else I
won't find my
equator

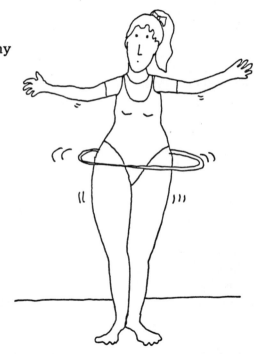

Remember when a Hula Hoop was a fad instead of a belt?

Building Fort Independence

Every time I pass up something I know I shouldn't eat, I am strengthening my defenses against overeating. I am fortifying myself against a food slip.

Just one "no, thank you," which turns aside a generous colleague coming at me with his bag of jelly-filled carbohydrates is enough to make me feel marvelous all day. I walk straighter. I have more energy. I even think with more clarity, since my brain is defogged of the guilt that follows overeating.

With every "no, thanks," I am building my freedom from a dependency on overeating. I am protecting myself against further assaults from food-pushers, like:
- Clients who appreciate the Big Lunch.
- Overhostly hosts and hostesses.
- Young vendors on my doorstep selling confections for some unquestionably worthwhile cause, usually during those after-school hours when my resistance sags.
- Hard-sell food merchants in stores or restaurants.
- Office co-workers who are bunny-eager to celebrate any and all occasions with pastries.

NO, THANK YOU.

I will practice this reaction until it becomes fully automatic. No, thank you, No, thank you, No, thank you. No, thank you. No, thank you. I will say it over and over again, out loud. A flimsy hand signal or a wag of my head will never convince ME that I mean it. I need to hear the firm, controlled, authoritative, no-buts-no-challenges sound of my own voice saying those wonderful, self-protecting words:

No, thanks.

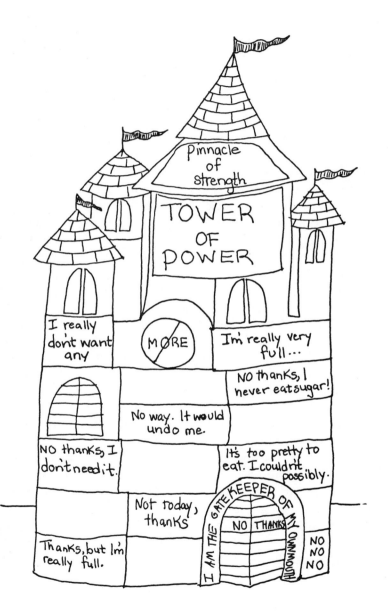

FATfalls: I shouldn't, but . . .

What is a FATfall? Every would-be thin knows. Call it a slip, a slide, a crash, a stumble, a splurge, a binge. We've all had them.

Generally, FATfalls seem to happen at three times:

1. At the half-hearted start of a weight-losing program, when we are not quite "with it" and our commitment to our thin selves is shaky.
2. When we are discouraged, our self-images are low, and we "don't care."
3. When we are euphoric with our losses to date.

The first two are entirely understandable. The last kind always comes as a shock. Why is it that when we think we are strong and have developed a resistance to temptations, when our admitted powerlessness over food (OA's First Step) seems to have been replaced by a feeling of Power and Control, when we are smug with success — that is the time we slip off our weight-losing programs. After a rosy week of dieting and losing, I find myself driving through the local food-through-the-window drive-in at 3:15 in the afternoon. What am I doing here? Just when I'm thinking, "Maybe I don't have an eating problem after all — maybe I've learned, finally, to overcome my compulsion," here I am, again.

After a No. 3 FATfall, I'm inclined to be discouraged and slip back into a No. 2 FATfall. Then my whole program deteriorates and I'm right back at No. 1.

Not every overweight has the same trouble with FAT-falls. Some fall harder. Some stay fallen longer. When we fall into our own built-in pillows, it's not so easy to pick ourselves up. Some — good for them! — are able to hop right back on the "abstinence" wagon with scarcely an upwards waver on the scale's pointer.

How can I head off a FATfall? By figuring out when and why it happens — what the precise situation is, what I am feeling at the time. Then bend over backwards (another cute trick for a FATso) to avoid a repetition. Sometimes it requires reorganizing my life to ignore clocks and calendars which have conditioned me to splurge at certain times.

By being aware at all times that I am, indeed, powerless over food, I can guard against a smug slide, a No. 3 FATfall. Haven't I proved that much to myself over and over again — every time I am pulled in off the street by a "Home Cooking" sign in a cafe window or a poster displaying the local Dairy Do's specialty in a container the size of a small skiff? Who's powerless? I am.

If I had a dime for every "I shouldn't, but . . . " that I've muttered, while *not* passing up what is passed on a plate, I could afford a winter at the Golden Door! Like most overweights, I set myself up for the crash. The only answer is to build my fortress of "no's." I am stronger with every refusal. I will also learn to skirt temptations. (Don't go by that magnetic fast-food place, with its cute soda fountain. Cross the street. Take another route.)

The following times, situations and states of mind — as reported in the fatalogues of several heavies — are standard pits for the portly:

365 birthdays a year

Somebody's birthday is always getting in the way of my diet. My birthday. My wife's, husband's, lover's birthday. My sister's and my cousin's and my aunt's birthday. My brother's, my mother's, my father's, my best friend's birthday. Or dozens of my acquaintances' birthdays. I could be celebrating someone-or-other's birthday every day of the year.

Suggestions: Unstick such notions as "I'll hurt Uncle Marvin's feelings if I don't eat a piece of his birthday cake" or "Mom will never get over it if I don't at least taste the one she baked for me." Uncle Marvin couldn't care less if you don't eat a piece; he'll just have an extra one left for tomorrow's lunch. And Mom will, too, get over it. You are the one who won't.

Borrow a quote from Marie Antoinette, with a slightly altered inflection: "Let THEM eat cake!"

Too little will during life's little ills

Is that old adage about feeding a cold still ringing in my head when my nose begins to stuff up? Funny, how I forget the second part of it, about starving a fever. Some of us OWs manage to remain ravenous even during an illness. One day of the green-apple two-step. and we are right back in the kitchen the next day — wan, but raring to eat. Our twenty-four-hour flu lasts a maximum of six or twelve. While mending from anything, from a lost appendix to a broken ankle, "keeping up my strength" means keeping up the extra weight along with it.

Suggestion: When you are sick, don't panic and go after food with all the desperation of a sinking person clutching a floating slat of shipwreck. If you have been getting along fine without refined sugar, don't blow it now for a sugary pop to "keep up my strength." Stay, whenever possible with your sensible eating plan. An occasional day of being unable to eat may be a positive poke in the direction of your weight-loss goal.

More aids for the "gotta eat when I'm sick" people:

_____

_____

_____

_____

The French-fried years

If I am a teen with a weight problem, I am shaping my future as well as padding my body. My prevailing attitude is: I care so much I have to act as though I don't care. With no difficulty at all, a teen can slip into the overeating habits of the Cruncher, the defiant one. I admit it is really tough to go along with the junk-food junkies and still be reasonable about my own eating. Besides, parents who help teens plan parties seem to assume that all teenagers are spaghetti or pizza freaks.

Suggestion: If you are feeling sort of rebellious anyway, start rebelling against the image of the all-American adolescent as a malt-slurper and French-fry-popper. Don't be embarrassed to take a Baggie full of carrot sticks to a movie or your own diet pop to a party. You may even start a trend. Keep the picture of yourself as a thin person, doing the things you like to do, stamped in your imagination. Don't let ups and downs of moods dictate what you eat. Avoid the crash that can follow a crash diet.

Get yourself — by bus, bike, car, family "taxi" service or foot — to a regular weigh-in program. Best of all, find yourself a weight-losing buddy and go together. Read the book, *Winning Weight Loss for Teenagers* by Joanne P. Ikena, R.D., Bull Publishing Co.

More ideas for the padded adolescent: _____

_____

_____

_____

Expanding the body along with the mind

If I am starting college, I am a candidate for a good case of freshman flab — that common condition especially prevalent on residential campuses which has parents and others close to the enlarging student doing double-takes at vacation times. How could Margie come home so suddenly round-faced and tight-jeaned? She is popping her rivets. Her hip-huggers are giving her bear hugs. Understandably, she is unhappy about herself.

The stresses of a new environment, scholastic pressures, a tinge of homesickness, institution food and probably a street full of escape-and-eat places — all these add up to a broadening experience.

Suggestions: Plan ahead. Limit your stops at local eateries, and don't fall into the practice of using them for study halls. Don't let munching-on-the-move become a habit. If you already have a weight problem, plan early to join a diet group or a diet table (or both). Don't abandon sports and exercise, now that you are spending hours sitting and studying.

I would avoid the freshman FATfall this way: _____

_____

_____

The pregnancy plumps

Nothing could be much truer than that oft-heard statement: If you don't put it on, you won't have to take it off. Prevention of overweight is key here, and your doctor is right to watch the scale. Probably the most clinging pounds many of us have collected are the ones gained during pregnancy and never unloaded.

If we were trees, you could count the number of our children by the number of layers, the rings in our cross-sections — a ring for every baby.

Failure to strip off the non-baby pounds once that wonderful baby is here may be caused partly by a shakeup in priorities and partly by an altered self-image. Of course, any new child is all-important. But check out that picture of self: Has it changed with the charge of motherhood — from girlish to mature, from spare to pillowy, from flat around the middle to roundish, from fast-moving to deliberate, from energetic to fatigued? Has Motherhood with a capital "M" so engrossed me that my own well-being has slid far down on my priorities list? Have I forgotten how to be selfish? At least selfish enough to keep my thinner goals in sight?

Though our children may be older now, we may still be plumped up with cushions from post-pregnancy FATfalls. Are we using the stresses and traumas of motherhood as an excuse for overweight?

Suggestion: One practical argument which can help you past the Martyrmom syndrome is to keep telling yourself that you are a healthier, better-adjusted, more realistic, more effective parent *without* the physical burden and the psychological complication of FAT. Besides, a thin parent probably will be around longer than a FAT one. Try this: I am a better parent when I am thinner (even *without* the after-school love offerings of home-baked cookies).

Add here any ideas you may have on how to keep from overgaining during pregnancy. _____

_____

_____

_____

Any ideas on how to regain — not regain, recover — your "as you were" status afterwards? _____

_____

_____

_____

Slowing down for the mid-stretch

Middle-agers often *expect* to spread. Although there may be changes in metabolism for women in the forties and fifties, they do not need to spell doom to the diet or an inevitable increase in breadth. Middle years, with their new freedoms, can mean a chance to grow without *growing*. Who said I had to slow down? (Borrow a little rebellion from the teen years here.) If I have been keeping up a regular program of exercise or an active sport, and if I have no medical reason to curtail my activities, why stop now? The middle-age spread is, mainly, in my head.

Suggestions: Keep up the exercise. Fill up your days — with a new career, a resumed career, new relationships, new challenges. Watch out for subtle changes in your lifestyle that may make these years in the middle add to your **own** middle. Are you walking less, driving more? Spending more time in culinary pursuits? Grandchild-sitting, which sometimes means, depending on the age of the grandchild, just that — sitting? Don't settle for adding pounds as you add years. This may be your liberated moment — the first breather in a long time that lets you take time out for yourself. Where is that thin self you have been promising yourself all these years? Now is the time to find it.

More cheers here for the middle years. How can you make them a time for positive thinning?

_____

_____

_____

_____

Clocks and calendars

If I take a minute to analyze FATfalls, I discover that the majority of them are governed by the clocks and calendars we live by.

Do I have trouble getting through a day without the five o'clock FATfall? Do I seldom make it through a year without the fall FATfall?

When the frost is on the pumpkin, I begin to look like one. If I live in a wintry clime, I — like my brother bruin — prepare to hibernate. The trouble is, that since I am not a bear, I don't actually hibernate. I just go right on preparing for it. Come spring, hibernation has pared down the bear, while I emerge from my winter coat noticeably unpared.

Weekends are the bottom for the always-on-Monday dieters. Somehow weekends are supposed to be special, fun-wise and food-wise. While we treat ourselves to rest and relaxation, fun and games, the pleasure of each others' company, we also treat ourselves to too much food.

Weekends are bad enough, but holidays are the very worst of the special, treat-yourself-to-food times. The

Curses on the ursus in us

When autumn comes I imitate
A bear about to hibernate
Who stuffs, then naps, and greets the spring much flatter.
But I'll always come to ruin by
Pretending I'm a bruin, I
Can never sleep it off, I just get FATter.

bigger the holiday, the bigger the spread (and ours). A groaning board, followed by the groanings of the too-full partakers, is the expected sequence on any given holiday.

I always needed at least a month to recover from Halloween. Guess who ate all the c-a-n-d-y the children collected in their trick-or-treat bags? My excuse? It was bad for *their* teeth!

Heavy Holidays

At Thanksgiving with our plump kin,
We dine on mince and pumpkin.
Will we ever learn to utter, "That's ENOUGH!"?
We're no sooner over this mistake
When extra pounds from Christmas make
Us know it's time for gobblers to unstuff.

In one way or another, we fight clocks and calendars our whole lives through. The following suggestions on how to keep clocks and calendars from being masters of our FAT fate, come from other overeaters:

Stay out of the kitchen at five o'clock. Pull your evening meal together earlier, at some non-hungry, non-stressful time of day, so you can warm it up during the pre-supper hour and not risk fussing with — and nibbling — ingredients.

About the fall FATfall? Monitor your weight with extra-ordinary vigilance. If autumn is your time for gaining, head into a serious weight-losing program instead. (Repeat to yourself: I am not a bear. I am not a bear. I am not a bear . . .)

As for weekends, try to treat Saturdays and Sundays like any other days. One former FAT we know spent unoccupied Saturday and Sunday hours at the office until he could look upon those days as ordinary, unspecial and not food-centered. Plan ahead for weekends, so you do not find yourself drifting in and out of the kitchen wondering what to do next. If the weather is decent, set outside chores for yourself — raking, gardening, painting. If home upkeep is not a concern, walk through a shopping center — briskly. Don't meander. Moving, not shopping, is your object.

A day is a day, and we get through it an hour at a time.

Holidays can still be times of togetherness, warmth and family feelings, without the usual overconsumption. Programs like Weight Watchers provide you with holiday dishes that are considerably lower in calories than the standard fare. Or forget the Big Holiday Dinner. What would happen if you invited your family or friends over for a turkeyless Thanksgiving musical or game of touch football? A cookieless, punchless Christmas caroling party? A hot-dogless Fourth of July turtle race?

How do you combat the tyranny of clocks and calendars? _____

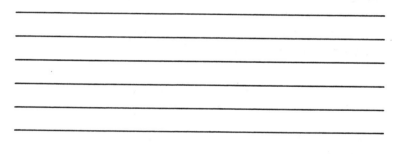

Eating out

If I am honest with myself, I really do not dread those chances to eat out, either at someone's house or in a restaurant. While outwardly sighing, "I don't know what I'm going to do about eating tonight, with all that good food around," I may be _looking forward_ to falling off my food plan. Perhaps I am not even conscious of how fast I clutch an excuse, while cloud-like visions of the host's favorite party dish or the restaurant's specialite de la maison waft to the top of my thoughts and hang there, tantalizing.

Now's the time for a pep-talk to self. "Self, you are

getting along just fine. You are beginning to see the outlines of your kneecaps and your ankle bones. You are beginning to sense the high of being thin, moving thin. No fancy dinner out on the town is worth the setback. Don't blow it."

Occasionally you may face a host or hostess who is piqued at you for ignoring the starchy casserole or refusing the Torte Splendide. But this situation is more rare than we like to think. And there are ways around it. If the invitation arrives by phone, don't be afraid to explain that you're really committed to a weight-losing program and you must partake sparingly.

If you need reinforcements, drag your doctor into it. "Doctor's orders" quell all manner of hostly protests. If a large group is invited, you can dish yourself a mountain of salad, spread it out over your plate, and the others will never know (until they run out of salad and trace the shortage to you).

As for the hostess and host who may be irked by your diet quirks — keep this in mind:

'Tis far better to offend 'em
Than to risk a FAT addendum.

About the restaurant scene . . . some of us do better eating out than fussing over the stove at home. Don't be shy about asking for broiled fish (hold the butter), salads (hold the goopy dressing) or whatever else fits in your plan. Most restaurant staffers are used to these special requests and will honor them as best they can.

Don't sit next to the case full of spinning desserts, or if you alight there by mistake, convince yourself that those dollops and wedges are made of cardboard and topped with plastic cherries. (It's only a paper prune cake, sailing around with a cardboard pie.) You'll be surprised at how you can convince yourself.

Know the menus of the restaurants you frequent and what they can do for you. If you are unsure about what they serve, call ahead and find out.

The parlors of temptation, the fast-food places, are

tougher to cope with. If other members of your family are drive-in-ophiliacs, compromise by eating the middles out of the wonders-in-a-bun. A shaved turkey, lettuce and tomato combination (hold the dressing, hold the bun) gets you by calorie-cheap.

Don't stay home and mope. The key is in the planning.

What techniques help you ensure that eating out will not destroy the continuity of your diet?

_____

_____

_____

_____

_____

Food shopping

This can be a daily FATfall, depending on how often I hit the supermarket. It has been said before. I will say it again, on the strength of personal experience. Don't food-shop on an empty stomach, unless you want to be lured by the siren songs emanating from every sugary item in the store. Shop only from a list. High noon (before lunch) and high teatime (before supper) are vulnerable moments.

Several of the FATfallen have admitted that, on the trip home from the market, the family car becomes a dining-room. (It's been everything else in this mobile age of ours!) Said one: "I used to eat in my car, so nobody could see me doing it." A head-in-the-sand fantasy, since an automobile is a rolling fishbowl. Anyone passing or approaching from the opposite lane can view clearly the working of the overeater's jaws, perhaps even the gleam of compulsion in the overeater's eyes. All very unbecoming for a FATtish person.

Are there crumbs in your glove compartment?
    Yes☐ No☐
Is your stick shift sticky? Yes☐ No☐

Are there dried apple cores under the foot pedals?
Yes☐   No☐

Such clues to FATfalls on wheels call for drastic rearrangement of food-shopping habits. Such as:

_____

_____

_____

_____

_____

_____

_____

_____

_____

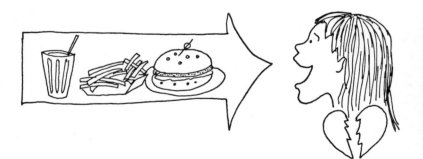

I eat because when I'm eating I don't have
to feel anything.

Humor Strategy

When you're at your desk or driving your car or riding a bus, just lift the corners of your mouth into the gentlest of smiles. And keep smiling. Even if you don't believe you're in the mood to laugh, feel the muscles in your body relax as you smile. Turning on a smile is like turning a valve to release tensions produced by stress.

Feel it? It's amazing. Besides, somebody might smile back — and that makes you feel even better.

Smile and you're halfway to a healthy laugh. Laugh, and you'll sense an easing of tension — the kind of tension that, unrelieved, can yank you like a magnet to food.

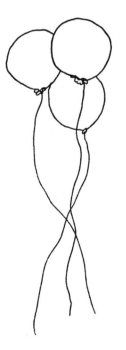

A Folk Song of the Resistance
(to the fast-food strip)

If fried fish and chips
Go right to your hips,
    Don't drive in,
    Drive on.

If a Big Burger bun
Makes you tons of NO-fun
    Don't drive in,
    Drive on.

If a Dairy Delicious
Is, for you, injudicious,
    Don't drive in,
    Drive on.

        If clams on the side
        Make you less tall than wide,
            Don't drive in,
            Drive on.

        If it's folly to eat those
        Bean-stuffed burritos,
            Don't drive in,
            Drive on.

        If Dixie fried chicken
        Is making you thicken,
            Don't drive in,
            Drive on.

If your extra flesh quakes
From those sixty-cent shakes,
   Don't drive in,
   Drive on.

If a pizza to go
Knocks you off your plateau,
   Don't drive in —
   Just keep right on moving, past all those twinkling
lights and deep-fried smells and dispensers of frozen dairy
products and carsful of skinny people parked with trays
propped on their windows. For you and for some of the
rest of us, the fast-food strip is a FAT-food trip.
   Drive on.

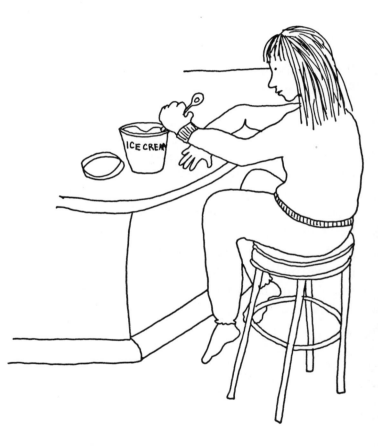

I eat because I feel empty all the time.

The stress that strains the seams

And here we have — in this corner — the toughest enemy of all for us thinning people, accountable for kayo-ing more diets and causing more FATfalls that any other hazard, including out-and-out hunger.

Some examples of FAT-producing stress:

One woman, mother of six, and her husband sold their house on the understanding that they would take possession of another. After weeks of on-and-off negotiations, the deal on the second house fell through. The toll: She gained back fifteen hard-lost pounds.

A pair of overweight parents added twenty pounds each while a son was in a treatment program (which involved them, too) for chemical dependency.

A middle-aged woman, caught in a crunch between adolescent children and aging parents, put on thirty while trying to make the decision to move her father to a nursing home.

Another woman, who had tried to cope with stress by drinking alcohol, overcame her alcoholism and found that she was using food for the same purpose. She had traded one dependency for another.

Other OWs have reported weight surges from a boggling variety of stresses — a particularly ragged divorce, a sick wife, an alcoholic spouse, a duel at work over who is going to win the race to the top, a daughter who has joined a cult or extremist movement, a waning sports career, crucial final exams, a job change, a husband's open-heart surgery, a nagging parent, a house fire, a barn fire, a first teaching job, a son in jail, a crippling accident, a depressed teenage child, loss of a beloved family pet.

The list, quite obviously, comprises some major, shattering, first-class stresses. But for some of us stress-eaters, it does not require any such severe trauma to set us off and eating. A minor stress — just some little niggling thing that unsettles us, that picks away at us, has exactly the same result: too much body. It can be a seemingly small matter:

- a phone call I dread to make;
- a shouting bout with a taxi driver;
- an unresolved argument with an offspring;
- a complaint from a neighbor;
- a dinky assessment for an interest charge from the Internal Revenue Service;
- an assignment to make an announcement to the PTA;
- a mislaid wallet;
- a lost earring;
- a haughty collection letter from a company which sent me my cancelled check two months ago;
- the unhappiness of a child who lost a swimming race;
- an unexpected call from the school principal;
- a lunch-date-time misunderstanding which left a friend waiting on a street corner;
- a "C" in a class I thought I had a "B" in;
- the disappearance of a pet rat in the chaos of a daughter's bedroom;
- the pain of a high school son's broken romance;
- a hotshot game of racquetball (or golf, or anything else) in which I play abominably.

Add five things here which are inclined to make you stress-eat. Identifying them is a large part of altering your behavior.

1. _____

2. _____

3. _____

4. _____

5. _____

Suggestions: Now that you have identified some of the reasons for your stress-eating FATfalls (you may not be conscious of them all, so the *Laugh It Off* chart at the back of the book on page 305 may find some others for you), the next move is:

1. To erase — or at least alleviate — the stresses from your life.

2. To learn new ways to handle them that don't involve popping food into your mouth.

Good luck with Number 1! Some stresses are just not erasable. Look back at your list of those five personal stress pits. Which ones can you eliminate?

Here is another "pinwheel": We overeat because we are reacting to the stress of overweight from overeating.

Number 2 here may be the greatest single aid to your living as a thin person.

Others have lessened their stresses — and also learned to control the overeating that can bring on added stress — through prayer, yoga, meditation, biofeedback, the Relaxation Response, centering, guided imagery, creative daydreaming, modeling (choosing someone to watch and emulate), role-playing, thought-stopping (yell "STOP!" every time you start to eat something you choose not to eat — or assign another person to yell it), and other popular means.

While exploring which of these methods might help you, try a little behavior change. Wait five minutes after the moment you feel compelled to run to the kitchen or the nearest food machine; see if the compulsion is still with you at the end of that "cooling off" period. That five-minute stretch may be an eon to you. Or it may be easy. In either case, it will begin to undermine your automatic reaction to stress — which is to EAT with all the frantic tide-stemming action of a crew sandbagging a rising river. The tide most of us seek to quell with too much food is our own roil of emotions.

You may have forgotten what stress-without-food *feels* like. Your response — to self-stuff — has been so trigger-automatic that you have not allowed yourself to feel what the stress is doing to you. Is it making you sad, frustrated, guilty, hurt, furious, anxious, frantic? If you are distressed, try to identify just *how* you are distressed. Once you discover how you feel, learn how to express it in appropriate ways. Overeating is not one of them.

When you feel a build-up of stress — say, it's a family hassle that makes you mad as a house cat left out in a rainstorm — substitute a walk around the block for your usual rush to the kitchen. You may not wear out all of that anger, but at least you will have found a new response (walking around the block) to the initial stress that used to send you ricocheting from refrigerator to cupboard to soft-drink closet.

Plug in here some substitute reactions to the most insidious FATfall of all — stress:

_____

_____

_____

_____

_____

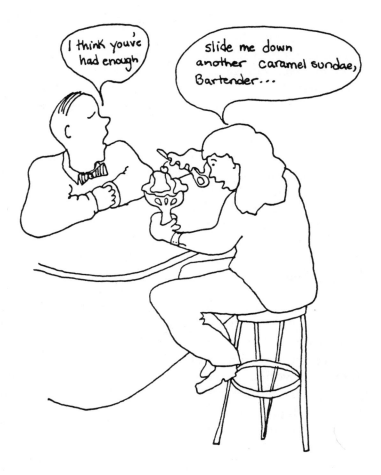

I eat because I don't drink.

Q. What is a FAT fantasy?

A. *A FATasy*

We overweight thin people remove ourselves so far from reality sometimes that we feed on the most elaborate illusions — along with too much food.

Among our FAT fantasies are these.

Do you ever indulge in the following self-soothing, self-fooling ideas?

FATasy No. 1: "Nobody notices how heavy I am," or the great FAT denial.

I can get by with lying about my weight to friends, family, drivers' license bureaus, the great hoodwinked public. I cannot lie to my doctor or my life insurance agent, though. Having to weigh in for either brings me back to the real world with a larger than average thud.

Tirelessly, I have researched the Big Cover-up. No one can determine my actual outlines because I hide them so well under the four-season navy-blue raincoat, baggy suits, a thundercloud of dark voile, or the various tents and awnings called caftans or mumuus or saris or kimonos, borrowed, in desperation, from other cultures.

Society plays right along with my own denial of my overweight with a hush-hush policy that comforts the FAT consumer with euphemisms, especially when it comes to covering unusual expanses of flesh with clothes. Because it might hurt my feelings and drive me away from clothing shops and back to the sewing machine, I am never — no, never — referred to as FAT, a word to be avoided tenderly.

I am "more woman," "twice as nice," "the mature figure" (even though I may be a mere age thirteen), an "elegant X," a "big and tall" man, a "plumpling" (coined by the founder of the National Association to Aid Fat Americans) or "queen-sized." How many FAT queens can you call to mind? England's Victoria might have been rather dumpy but, generally, regality and queenliness are not synonyms for FAT.

Society never confronts me openly by saying, "You, there, you're FAT." If I deny my FAT facts, everybody else will gloss over my weight problem, too. Only when I choose to open my eyes do I see that I really live in a thin world, that it is neither fashionable nor healthy to be overweight. Under my layers of denial, if I am really honest with myself, I can recognize that the same thin world is telling me, in a thousand sideways ways, to shape up. I am the abnorm, the outsize, the misfit.

I can change all that.

FATasy No. 2: "Somewhere, sometime there will be an instant-thin plan, pill or potion."

I might as well wait until the Great Discovery. Then I will be able to lose the extra pounds with no effort on my part, through some miracle. Actually, our own minor miracle will be losing the extra weight, which is — by all statistics — shortening our lives.

FATasy No. 3: "FAT is just a matter of timing."
I will lose it when (check any that apply to you):
☐ I shed my baby FAT
☐ my life becomes less stressful
☐ I get rich and can buy better food
☐ I stop having children
☐ my children are all in school
☐ I find someone I can really care about
☐ I get a raise and can join a health club
☐ I can leave the farm with its big-eating atmosphere
☐ I can get out of the restaurant business
☐ I retire and can concentrate on myself for a change
☐ I feel better — it's so hard to diet when I'm sick
☐ I graduate and get away from this starchy, institution food

Other time-is-never-right fantasies: _____

_____

_____

FATasy No. 4: "No one close to me really cares whether I'm FAT or not. After all, it's *my* body."

Or, taking it a step further: "My husband doesn't care. He just says I'm 'more to love.' " Retort from the Voice of Reality: Woman, if he cares about you, he'll wish for *less* to love. He will want you thinner, healthier and longer-lasting.

I interpret a family member's silence on the subject of my weight as don't-care, when actually that person may realize — rightly — that nagging accomplishes nothing. Yes, it is, after all, my body. And I am the only one who can change what gravity does to me. Just because my friends and family don't talk about my extra pounds does not mean that they overlook them. Anyone who loves me wants me healthy. FAT, I am definitely not as healthy as I could be.

Our FAT fantasies may also be FAT rationales — reasons why we find ourselves in our present state of overweight. Most of them are unreasonable reasons, which put them in the category of fantasies. Some of the more common why's for heaviness, usually offered in all solemnity, are these:

FATasy No. 5: "It's my glands. They don't seem to work like other people's." Studies show that a small percentage — perhaps one in twenty — of all heavies have any kind of glandular or other physical disorder which could be a significant cause of overweight. It's my glands, all right — my salivary glands!

FATasy No. 6: "It runs in the family."

An overweight (OW) points to a mother, father, sister, brother, aunt, cousin, grandmother, as evidence of a family-wide case of the FATs. The question is: Is the corpulence of kin the result of a hereditary tendency, or more often of family eating and exercise habits.

FATasy No. 7: "I'm so nervous all the time."

A lot of people are nervous, but not all are overweight.

The large person giving this excuse may not have explored other ways of handling stress or developed any necessary spiritual strengths. This person is using food as a tranquilizer — a regular practice among overweights. (Sugar actually is a chemical tranquilizer, according to Dr. Irwin Lublin, a California State University at Los Angeles psychologist, known also for aversion therapy, who has completed an eight-year study on weight control.) Perhaps we do learn to depend on sugary tranquilizers, and we bulge accordingly. The fantasy is that *because I am nervous, I must also be overweight.* Not true. And such a negative thought may be an obstacle to growing thin.

FATasy No. 8: "I can't lose because I retain water." (Or, for women, "because I'm on the pill.")

Here is the old water-weight ploy. It is true that women do have to cope with pre-menstrual bloat, and "water pills" have been known to nudge us off a plateau and onto a losing path again. But if we lean too heavily on *both* the water pills *and* the excuses, without altering our eating habits, we can get stuck. Heavies who cling to the idea that "we don't need to diet — all we need is to take a diuretic and the weight will go away" have sometimes been trapped on not just a plateau, but the Great Plains.

In any case, such medication should be taken only if a doctor prescribes it. Your doctor can give you suggestions on how to get over your "I can't lose" fantasy, probably starting with reducing your salt intake, or adding such natural diuretics as parsley or asparagus or cider vinegar to your diet. Don't forget such overlooked sources of salt as diet soft drinks.

Fluid retention can be a cause for discouragement, but does not have to turn you into a gorging defeatist. There are ways to break out of the monthly gain-and-lose-only-to-gain-again pattern.

The greatest "water problem" for men and women alike, involves our own hydraulics — and the mechanism that pivots on the elbow and carries the hand and forearm in a sweeping ninety-degree arc from table to mouth!

FATasy No. 9: "When I am sick, I need more food." (See also under FATfalls.)

With "feed a cold" (I practically never have a "starve a fever" problem) replaying in my head for the umptieth time since toddlerhood, I eat to "feel better." When a certain food does not seem to improve my health, I try another — and another — and another. Any symptom at all is an excuse to abandon my diet plan. If I have given up refined sugar, I use sickness as an excuse to glom onto the nearest sugar-coated, sugar-filled item for comfort. As I am an avowed, genuine, sticky-fingered sugarholic, this sends me skidding into a binge.

Any other FATasies? Record them here: _____

_____

_____

_____

_____

_____

_____

_____

FAT myth:

Everyone burns calories
at the same rate.

FAT truth:

An OW burns more calories than a
thin person for the same amount of
exercise. (It takes more to move us
around.)

FATtraps

Have I taken on a permanent role which keeps me in a forever-FAT trap?

☐ **The "such a good cook!" role.** Because I have a reputation for being a culinary wizard, I spend hours in the kitchen producing wonders to uphold the gourmet standards I have set for myself. Cooking is my claim to distinction, and also my road to EXtinction. Somewhere during my history in the kitchen, I made the switchover from gourmet to gourmande (from one who appreciates fine cuisine to one who gluttonizes). I now need a new way to distinguish myself — outside the kitchen — this may take some explaining to my food fans. I may have to swallow a little pride instead of my own creative cuisine. But it is worth it.

☐ **The "gourmet" role.** This is the consumer end of the culinary arts department. I have made myself an authority on fine dining, fine wines, fine restaurants. Like the creator of wondrous edibles (above), I, the knowledgeable consumer, have an image to preserve. I am, at the same time, preserving body FAT. It is time to take on a new field of study, to cancel my subscription to *Haute Cuisine* (or the equivalent) and pick up *Weight Watchers* magazine instead. It is time to avoid those fancy restaurants, until I can learn how to order thinning fare. It is time to picture myself in a new, thin role.

☐ **The Big Guy or "big enough for my boots" role.** (Also see the Big Eater, one of the Classic Overeaters.) This one results in executive bloat. I am the Big Guy who can eat anything, drink anything, take on anybody — and win. Somehow bigness and authority and machismo and leadership are all related for me. I think in terms of Big People in Big Positions. But I am beginning to bog down from bigness. When I no longer swagger from choice, but from necessity, I need to rethink. Brawn is okay. Tough is okay. Big is not.

☐ **The Mighty Mom role.** In my mind — as in the mind

of the Big Guy — "big" and "strong" match up. It is not so bad being heavy when you can lift your weight in furniture. It is useful for a mother to be able to hoist an old dresser up an apartment stairwell or a one-hundred-and-ten-pound sheepdog onto a vet's examining table. I have never been known to turn down a challenge to lug, tote, spade, shovel, wheelbarrow anything at ground level. (I avoid ladders.) But lately my face gets redder and my breathing noisier than they once did during such undertakings. Mighty-Mom-to-the-rescue needs rescuing herself — from her mighty FATtrap.

☐ **The "eat-everything teen" role.** Even though this is a temporary role limited to teen years, it can take its toll in extra rolls around the belt line. My thinking goes something like this: All teens munch out. (I will, too.) All teens hang around fast-food places. (I will, too.) All teens eat everything in sight. (So will I.) The truth is, some teens don't. Some only *pretend* to go along with the munch-out-bunch. If I can just find some other kids my own age who don't believe in the eat-everything (or the try-everything) idea . . .

☐ **The "helpless" role.** I am a pudgy puppet of circumstance. I do not act. I react. I count on those around me to make my decisions, explanations, explorations. I don't even know how to have my own fun. Naturally, my helplessness extends to my eating. I probably am *supposed* to be FAT. God must have intended me to be a FAT person. My only way out of the helpless hole begins with taking responsibility for my *self*, including my heft.

☐ **The "I am unique" role.** Well, I am, of course, so this is an entirely defensible statement. But as a role for the would-be-thinner, it's a snag. It brings on this sort of self-talk: Since I am special, I do not have to follow the prescribed food plan. I can mix and match at will, taking one food idea from one diet, one from another, counting calories here, leaning heavily on a certain kind of food there. (Naturally, diets are put together to be exclusive, to stand alone, without substitutions, elaborations or additions. Mixing-and-matching is an unnecessary exercise in creativity which gets me nowhere.)

The "I am unique" idea applied to losing weight sometimes can be a real diet-stopper. "I don't lost weight like other people do; I can starve and not lose an ounce." Such negatives can bomb all the motivation I may have mustered.

A corollary of "I am unique" is "I can do it myself." While there are those, the superdedicated, who can take off the extra pounds all on their own, it is a lot easier, more fun, less lonely to find a group or a weight-counselor or a doctor who regularly treats overweight patients. I need someone else to say, "Wow," as the pounds drop, or to explain the now-and-then slight upwards flicker of the scale indicator.

☐ **The "if I can't be perfect, I won't try at all" role.** Starve or stuff. I am always judging myself and finding that I don't measure up to my steep standards of perfection. If I can't be the most magnificently proportioned body of all time, I won't try for a respectably proportioned body. If I can't be a superlative wow, I'll be a cow. This is a copout of the first degree. I need to strive for the best I can be (which is better than I think). Skip the comparisons.

☐ **The "at home at the range" role.** The symbol of home (in my own mind, at least), is not the hearth, cozily exuding warmth and familyness, it is I, myself, planted firmly and FATly in front of the stove — ready at all times to feed and provide. Even though I may have a job somewhere else, too, my heart is not in it. I am, first of all, a home body (a home *big* body). I relish my image as the core of the household, the fixed center around which all family activity spins. I am the puffed-up mother bird (I could be a grandmother bird, or an aunt bird, or a father bird and still play this role), prepared to nourish not only my own fledglings, but any other strays who happen to perch temporarily on the rim of my nest. In times of crisis, I comfort — with food. I distract — with food. I humor — with food. I am the ample, parently lap. If that lap becomes any ampler, it may vanish altogether. How can I possibly leave my central post — at home at the range? Perhaps I have not heeded as seriously as I might have the feminist outcries that have fallen upon my ears. Perhaps I had better listen and develop some interests of my own — just for me. The alternative may be a case of the empty-nest FATS.

What other roles do you find yourself stuck in, for which FAT, stereotypically, is an appropriate costume? What other FATitudes about yourself are traps which resist change and keep you in the too-much-flesh category?

_____

_____

_____

_____

_____

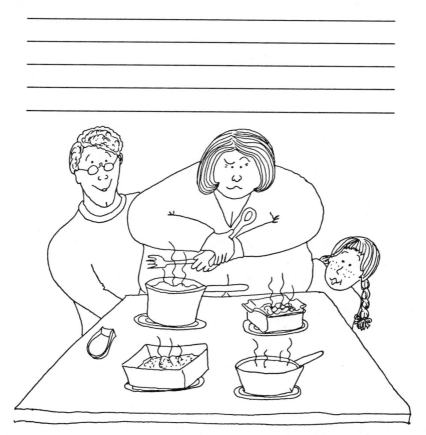

"My spoon rest doesn't see a lot of action."

The fitting-room fits

At some time or other, all of us OWs need to cover our bodies, if not fashionably, at least appropriately. That means facing that cold island of truth — the fitting room.

I sneak into the cubicle with three sizes of slacks over my arm: 1) the least possible size (large); 2) the slightly more possible size (larger); 3) the "Oh-no-it-can't be" size (huge).

On the way to humiliation, the glacial eye of a suspicious salesperson catches mine, as she mistakenly interprets my stealth as an attempt at shoplifting. I am overcome by the double injustice of such a gaze. Not only do I read in it, "You are FAT," but also, "You are a FAT thief."

I rush, sweating and purple-faced, hair wild and sticky with electricity, to cover my body before the same salesperson whips aside the curtain or bores a fishy glance at me through a louver.

Yank on one pair of slacks. Impossible. Teeter out of that pair. Yank on another. Teeter out of those. Try again. Armholes make almost-ripping sounds as I attempt to time my body-baring with the salesperson's absence. A zipper sticks or runs off its trolley from sheer strain. I, of course, have to confess it. The salesperson sighs.

When she asks the inevitable, "How were they?", I have the nearly uncontrollable urge to screech, "None of your business!" (even though it obviously *is*), while returning all three sizes with polite murmurings about how they "weren't quite what I had in mind."

I may emit a whoop akin to a primal scream, all politeness blown away, if just one more clothing sales type refers to "slimming lines" or "larger" sizes. As if the comparative "larger" were somehow less damning than the simple (and true) "large." Larger than what? Larger than normal? If one more salesperson clears the fitting room of my rejects with a "poor FAT you" air of exasperated defeat, I may never try on another stitch. Oh, the haughtiness of the superstylish thin!

To avoid the physical exertion and the wear and tear on our psyches, some of us have resorted to buying our mix-and-don't-bother-to-match separates from tables of rumpled sale items. Just grab the largest size and hope. Take them home, untried. How many of us have closets full of such casual purchases, most of which don't come close to fitting us? With a shape that changes as often as the weather, we may fit almost any of these rags sometime.

For me with the extra, the fitting-room becomes a crucible of self-deprecatory feelings. It is also the supreme court which judges the extent of my FATness. I am the judge, I am the jury, I am the defendant. I am guilty of FAT in the third degree. (Easy there, FAT is not a crime.)

The value of the fitting-room fits, painful as they are, is that they are a lesson in reality. Here I stand, half-stripped, under relentless fluorescent lights, caught between two mirrors, with truth shining at me fore and aft. I am, honestly appraised, a creature of epic proportions and unclassy dimensions. My lines are not smooth. They ripple, indent, fold over. I would be a hard one to follow the dots around.

It is time — the mirrors, the lights, the size numbers on the tags, the salesperson's condescending attitude tell me so — to change for the thinner.

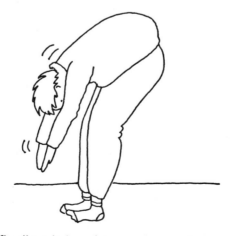

Am I finding it hard to make ends meet?

Humor Strategy

Delight in funny sounds. Extremes of instrumental highs and lows. Children laugh at the blurt of a tuba or silvery pourings from a piccolo. Synthesizers have a vocabulary of humorous sounds.

Listen for new and funny noises that can make you laugh.

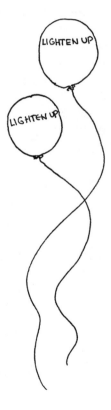

When is spreading myself too thin spreading myself FAT?

Am I too busy to get thin? Am I caught in the density and variety of events — the helter-skelter push-push of schedules, meetings, obligations, niceties, celebrations? If I am a person who gets FAT on complications — and a lot of us are — the answer is yes. Along with complications come anxieties, and along with anxieties come pounds.

For some of us who wear not one, not two, but six or seven hats in a day, life is far from serene. We are a society of multiple-hat-donners.

With every hat-switch, we have to change our pace, our mood, our style, even our clothes. We are putting on stage productions with limited casts, in which each one of us plays several totally different parts. We have become experts at the quick change in the wings.

We have overloaded ourselves not only with job and household commitments, but with a succession of desperate causes — save our elms, save our morals, save our educational standards, save our gas.

The geographical breadth of our activities requires every kind of craft from superjet to moped. Our too-full calendars are so solid with scribbles that we need a speedy-reading course in order to make it through a single week. No week-at-a-glance for us!

Because people are living longer (especially thin people), we are caught up in the responsibilities of four-generation families. Divorces have presented some of us with two pairs of parents, sometimes even an extra grandparent-come-lately or two. Though we are grateful for loving relatives, just keeping up with a host of them can be a consuming matter.

The result of spreading ourselves too thin? We have spread ourselves FAT. The working-wife-mother has become a well-rounded woman. The man of many roles has turned into a man of many rolls. The overscheduled teen chunk flees from life's demands into a vinyl oasis of peace at the neighborhood Stuff 'n Sip — and stuffs and sips.

Rate the following activities in their order of importance to you. (Number 1 is the most important, 2 less important, and so on.) In the second column, rate them again, according to the amount of your time each requires. (Number 1 takes the most time, 2 less time, and so on.)

General activity	Importance to you	Time spent
Furthering your education (classes, seminars, workshops)	_____	_____
Furthering your career (working at a job, profession)	_____	_____
Being a wife (husband)	_____	_____
Being a loving partner	_____	_____
Parenting	_____	_____
Taking care of household needs (cooking, washing, cleaning, repairs)	_____	_____
Chauffeuring children	_____	_____
Helping care for other relatives	_____	_____
Being a concerned citizen of your community	_____	_____
Engaging in active sports	_____	_____
Engaging in spectator sports (from Little League to bigger league)	_____	_____
Pursuing arts (music, dance, theater, art — either as artist or viewer)	_____	_____
Meeting spiritual needs (church, synagogue or other)	_____	_____
Traveling	_____	_____
Entertaining or otherwise socializing for business reasons	_____	_____
Entertaining or socializing for nonbusiness reasons	_____	_____
Keeping in touch with people (telephoning, writing letters)	_____	_____

Add here any others that occur to you. Rate them in the same way.

General activity	Importance to you	Time spent
_____	_____	_____
_____	_____	_____
_____	_____	_____
_____	_____	_____
_____	_____	_____
_____	_____	_____
_____	_____	_____
_____	_____	_____
_____	_____	_____

Does this tell you anything about yourself?

Now list the specific activities that crowd your life (PTA, choir, committees, job, evening school, bowling team, golf, herpetology club, investment club, unusually burdensome household task). Again, prioritize these pursuits and rate them according to how they eat up your time. If you list six or more, what would happen if you dropped all those extra extras that are least important to you?

Specific activity	Importance to you	Time spent
_____	_____	_____
_____	_____	_____
_____	_____	_____
_____	_____	_____
_____	_____	_____

Would paring down your schedule help you pare?

How can you organize your time to avoid a FAT frenzy? How can you avoid spreading yourself FAT?

Unhooking the super-caloric combos

Another key, a master-skeleton key to help us find our own skeletal armatures under all the blub:

When you eat, just eat. Don't combine eating with other activities.

Some of us are the busy-busy kind who need to do a minimum of two things at once. We eat *and* look at television, eat *and* gabble on the telephone, eat *and* listen to music, eat *and* write a letter, eat *and* sit in a movie theater, eat *and* work at a desk.

I need to discover what my eating is twinned with — and then unhook the combination. I must have enlarged my body with hundreds of thousands of unconsciously consumed calories while I was doing something else along with eating.

Gobblewatching: Eating and looking at TV

Eating *and* watching television are the most perilous pair of all for the serious FATfighter. This team of arch villains probably is responsible for more excess poundage than any other twinned activities. The fact that we are presently a nation of watchers instead of doers, observers instead of performers, has a direct bearing on our national (and individual) problem of overweight. Simply put, we sit more than we ever did in ages past — when we had to haul water, split wood, grow our own food and cover more territory on foot. And most of our sitting is in front of the television screens. We plahtz there. Or, even less energetically, we lie there, prone with our heads propped, spaced out on the hum from the TV set.

If we move at all, it is back to the kitchen for replenishment inspired by a food commercial.

We dine, plates on knees, before the television. (Another few centuries of this sort of sedentary viewing, and we'll develop flattened knees and laps like table tops.)

We pre- and post-dine with one hand clutching food, the other on the channel selector.

Ask us what we have eaten? We never know.

If gobblewatching is so ingrained in our scheme of living that unhooking TV from eating seems impossible, it may be necessary to give up television for a while. Let's, for our thin selves' sake, by all means remove the TV set from the kitchen, if that's where it is. If I have to do something else while watching television, I will hook a rug or wood-carve. And I will tune out the commercials that glamorize foods and perk up my too-responsive appetite.

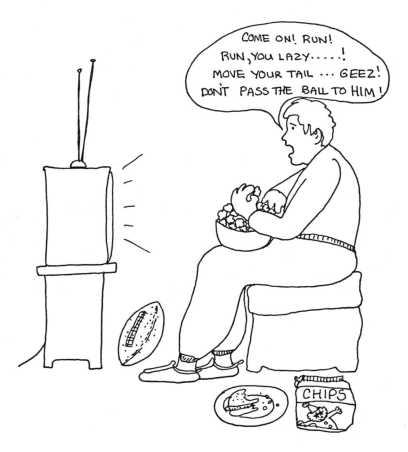

Moviemunching: Eating at the movie theater

Food bought in the theater lobby is usually staggeringly expensive and abundantly caloric. Such vendors rarely provide so much as a sugar-free drink for those of us who care. Some of us cannot go to a movie without purchasing and passing around a bucket of buttered popped stuff. And who is it that chooses to harbor the reach-in bucket? Whose lap is bucket headquarters? Who ends up with the most buttery fingers?

If I have moviemunching written indelibly into my script, I will fill up with a big salad before I hit the cinema lobby with its confection counter and popping-machine. Or I will take along an apple, or sugarless gum. Sometimes it is easier to substitute an allowed food item than it is to remove the food altogether. And I will kick the bucket habit. I will let somebody else, at the other end of the row, hold it.

Puffeating: Eating and smoking cigarettes

Dealing with twin compulsions at once could require another entire book's worth. A cigarette between courses of a meal seems to "make more room." A big meal makes a cigarette "taste better," so the smokers say. Read some of the many books available for ideas on how to give up smoking and not turn into a non-smoking blimp from overeating.

For those so desperate about their weight that they consider turning to — or returning to — smoking cigarettes, we have a word: Don't. Puff the Magic Wagon is not the magical, easy-to-stay-on food-abstinence wagon you may expect. While smoking seems to help satisfy an oral compulsion, you end up with two addictions instead of one — food and cigarettes. If you do not already have these twin compulsions, for heaven's sake (and yours) do not acquire them. It means double trouble — perhaps even double doom.

Phonefilling: Eating and talking on the telephone

The telephone cord that stretches to the refrigerator can be well-nigh umbilical. How often do I find myself reaching for something to eat when the phone rings — or when I have to make a phone call that I dread? Phone rings. Left hand holds receiver. Right hand goes automatically to the latch on the refrigerator or the button on the breadbox or the knob on the cupboard door. I have become adept at opening a cracker box one-handed. I have learned to chew oh-so-silently, alternating munches with mumbles, in order to hide my phonefilling from the person on the other end of the line.

Some practical answers: Move the telephone to a place in the house that is far from the food supply. Shorten up the stretch cord on the telephone. (That twelve-footer was installed when the kids were little and I needed to survey four rooms while on the telephone. Now that they are past the age when I need to umpire their actions, a six-foot line will do just as well.) Save any long-winded calls and make them from a foodless area, like a phone booth. What it saves in calories may be worth the quarter.

Other eating-and's that need uncoupling

Eating *and* studying, or eating *and* reading. Are there food smudges on the pages of every good book on your shelves? An apple-and-a-book are a classic combination, that is not excessively FAT-making, unless you are into a 600-page book and you require an apple for every fifty pages. That totals twelve apples and approximately 1,000 calories per book. If you are an apple-and-bookworm, try reading in the local library, which usually is snackless.

Eating *and* drinking. A cocktail party can be a dieter's demise. Most of us are acknowledged foodaholics, and some of us may even be recovering alcoholics, turned foodaholic. A compulsion is a compulsion, and all of the "holics" seemed to be related. The drinking man's (woman's) diet aside, one drink makes me want to eat. Or rather, it makes me not care how much I eat. If I am serious about losing weight — and this time, I am — I will cut out the occasional cocktails and all the pretty little dinner wines and any before- and after-dinner drinks. They add sugar, and they add calories. If I have caloric limitations, I would rather eat the calories than drink them anyway.

Eating and balancing the checkbook

Recognize this still life? Calculator. Checkbook. Pen. Plate of food. Mug of coffee (or some other drink). This caloric combo — for me — stems directly from the food-is-a-reward misdefinition. I am being so *good* to sit down and do this dull task, one of life's boring necessities. Therefore I deserve a simultaneous food treat. In this case, figures do not help me regain mine.

Certain eating and's are occupational hazards for dieters

Take writing. The stock portrait of the writer is the writer-*and*-smoker. Hail-like flurries of typing followed by thoughtful draws on the cigarette. I give you another: the writer-*and*-eater. Hail-like flurries of typing followed by thoughtful swallows of food. Occasional — perhaps frequent — leaps up to run to the kitchen, presumably in search of a word, a phrase, an idea. Return to the typewriter without the apt phrase, but with a handful of food instead.

Then, of course, there is the salesman or account executive who uses fancy restaurants as client-bait and, not surprisingly, turns into a whale in the process. Eating *and* client-polishing.

There are the busy, on-their-feet people — salespersons, waiters and waitresses — for whom sitting and eating is synonymous with peace, a break in the day's activities. The business "break" means a coffee break, which usually means a coffee-and-goodie break. Eating *and* taking time out.

Truckers who roll from one good-food truck stop to

another eat according to fine old-fashioned he-man (or she-woman) standards. "Off the road" means "at the food counter." But the calories used up in driving a truck down a highway do not match the caloric input. Result: A hefty breed of truckdrivers. Eating *and* driving.

Others in a sitting society have similar problems: police officers who patrol in a car (squad seat), bus drivers (bus butt), secretaries and office workers (secretarial spread), taxi drivers (cab flab), operators of sewing machines (seamstress — or seamster — beam). And these comprise only a sample.

Add other occupational eating-*and* hazards here. There are plenty of them:

Even more specifically, certain foods seem to belong with certain situations. Peanuts *and* circuses. Popcorn *and* movies. Hot dogs *and* baseball games. Turkey *and* Thanksgiving. Potato salad *and* Fourth of July. Ham *and* Christmas. The after-the-movie stop at the soda fountain. The après-swim cone. The after-church pancakes. (Read this paragraph fast and go on to the next without dilly-dallying.)

Social snarfing* or team-eating

The destructive combinations of eating-*and's* may include other food-snarfing people. For me, it is much more important to escape from a social wolfer than a social wolf. These snarfers may be FAT, thin or in between. They may be acquaintances, kin, lovers, business associates or longtime buddies. To zero in on my weight-losing project, I may have to unhitch myself, firmly and decisively, from these overeating types, especially at mealtime — or at any of the random times of day or night they choose to go snarfing.

A friendly Binge-eater may catch me up in the devil-may-care abandon of regular splurges. Preambles to watch out for: "C'mon, let's go out and get a _____" or "Gee, the Flying Dutch Horse is still open and I'm hungry for a _____" or "Take a break. You deserve it. How about a _____?"

A visiting Nibbler and I, when teamed, can swoop through the larder like a buzz of locusts, laying waste to all that's ingestible.

At work, even though the sound comes from across the room, a Cruncher's chomping may turn me on to whatever crunch-foods are being shared that day. Typically, Crunchers keep crackling bags of chips and other noisies in their lockers or desk drawers. I may have to move myself out of earshot.

If I share a coffee break regularly with an overeater, one who falls predictably for the sweetpuff or the glazed whatsis, I find temptation tapping at my very elbow. My daily rut of going out for lunch with the same overeater(s) contributes to my downfall. I had better look for alternatives — a walk down the avenue, a workout at a close-by spa or YWCA or YMCA, a window-shopping trip, a quick once-over at a museum exhibition.

Planning ahead and brown-bagging a lunch gives me the control I need.

---

*to snarf: a particularly apt term, perhaps a regionalism, meaning to ingest large quantities of food with abandon.

If I am a weight-aware teenager, social snarfing is an especially acute problem. If I care enough, I will keep away from munch-everything-in-sight peers and look for a friend who is as determined as I am to take off the padding.

But what do you say to someone with whom you have been co-indulging at lunch or at an after-school sweets stop for months, even years?

Be honest. "I am serious about losing weight this time — serious enough to change my habits drastically." Take your doctor's name in vain if you must. Suggest alternatives for spending time with your fellow splurger, activities that do not involve food.

Strategies to keep your friends your friends and your relatives your relatives while breaking away from FAT-building patterns of co-eating or team-eating:

_____

_____

_____

_____

_____

_____

_____

_____

_____

_____

_____

_____

_____

_____

_____

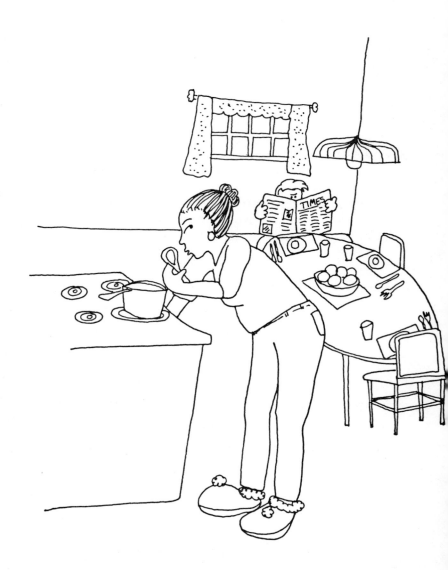

Calories don't count if you're only "tasting"

My misery is bigger than your misery

An OW man thinks:

Women have it all over men when it comes to overweight. An overweight woman, unless she is grossly overweight, still is considered "soft" and "feminine." But for a man to be thought of as FAT — and therefore "soft" — destroys the fine, tough, lean-bodied image he regards as standard for the American male. Doughiness is a threat to his masculinity. Besides, a woman can wear some sort of a filmy tent to cover herself.

An OW woman thinks:

An overweight woman has a much harder time than an overweight man. There is no such thing as a "FAT man." Only women are regarded as "FAT." Men are just "big." Besides, a man can hide his bigness in a baggy suit, while a woman is expected now and then to bare an arm or a shoulder or an ankle or two. If what is bared is FAT, her appeal drops like the temperature in International Falls in January (along with her self-image). An obese woman falls into a classification of "repulsive," while an obese man is simply a sort of teddy bear character. Besides, girl babies ordinarily have more built-in FAT cells in which to store FAT for the rest of their lives. And men, once they make the decision to lose, can take off the weight faster.

Who wins?

When it comes down to comparisons, nobody — no large body — male or female comes out on top.

Is the skeleton in your family closet a FAT body?

(Your own?)

Is FAT a family disease?

More and more weight-losing plans involve the thin members of the family, along with the would-be-thinner. A dieter does not diet in a vacuum, but in an environment that includes one or more other humans sitting around — or walking around — eating things. It also includes a larder usually well laden with whatever it takes to feed whoever else lives there.

The "after all, it's MY body" FATitude holds up if I'm living in a cave in the side of a mountain with nothing but pet hyenas for company. (Even *they* might chortle over my FAT plight.) But if I am living with people, as part of a twosome or a family or a group, my pounds weigh on those others, too. Why else should I be so guilty about my overweight? Comments like these are avenues for truth:

"I beat up (note: translate as "got beat up by") a sixth-grader on the school bus who said, 'Your Mom looks like a football player.' "

"Can you imagine Dad in a canoe?" (followed by tittering.)

"I have to stay home to help Sis paint the living-room. We don't dare let her climb on a stepladder."

"I thought I was taking on *one* woman when I got married. Now it's more like two!"

"The best seats are up high, but we can't ask Uncle Bert to crawl up in those bleachers. He might fall through."

"I went to six stores looking for a sweater big enough

for Grandma, and I couldn't find one."

"Mom, if you hadn't let out your wedding dress after you gained all that weight, I could have worn it."

"Other Dads go skating with their kids. But Dad says if he fell down he'd break the rink."

Whether I admit it or not, my extra weight does affect those close to me. My family members may be hiding me, making excuses for me, forgetting (on purpose) to pass on invitations or challenges because they know I cannot participate. They may be hounding me about my weight, or they may be hushing up the whole subject for fear of bruising my feelings. Whatever their reactions to my problem, I am not an isolated person in a padded cell. I — along with my extra FAT — am interrelating with everyone close to me.

This awareness need not bog me down with guilt. Just let it be an added impetus for a thin transformation.

I will not be too proud or secretive to ask my family for help during my program for change. If I am a woman with household responsibilities, my request might sound something like this:

"I take full responsibility for my own weight loss. Whatever pounds I have put on, I can also take away. But I need your support and your understanding, even though you may be inconvenienced now and then.

"Please help me cut my time spent in the kitchen to a minimum. Please don't ask for the kind of meals that keep me there puttering in elaborate preparations. Please understand that, for now, there will be no baked desserts or sweet scoops or snacks in the refrigerator or cupboards. If you must have these, please eat them away from home — at least until I have developed the discipline to resist them.

"Please understand when I turn down certain invitations involving food. Please do not expect me to go out to restaurants that cannot accommodate my kind of eating.

"Please do not ask me how the diet is going, or about how much weight I have lost. Please do not tease, nag or scold me, laugh at me or act as my conscience. Let me do these things myself — for myself.

"Please understand that, at least for now, my first priority is my own commitment to lose weight. It has to take precedence over job, friends, marriage and parenthood. If it seems to be a selfish project, it is because it must be in order to succeed.

"I need your encouragement and your understanding. I need your agreement that my weight-losing is a worthwhile effort.

"You cannot take the pounds off my body for me, but you, my beloved(s), can help me keep on caring."

Some programs supply their weight-losers with a "Letter to Families" enlisting their support. Other diet programs, too, are recognizing that families count when you are trying to countdown for a weight loss.

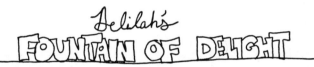

GRUNT BURGERS• SLIDERS• SALTED DOO-DAHS

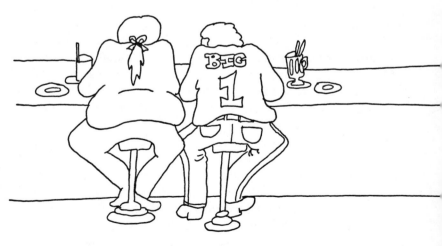

Chewing the fat

Saboteurs, mostly unwitting

Just a few words about saboteurs. Not many words, because I might catch myself right back in the midst of my FAT trick of blaming. Who are those rock-hearted villains who undermine in subtle ways my earnest efforts to trim? Usually those close to me, within my family or in my clutch of friends. Most often they are unaware of what they are doing, but I do need to be aware of them, on guard and ready to retaliate, if necessary.

Some standard models of saboteurs:

The husband or wife, openly campaigning for the spouse's weight loss, who becomes the loser's conscience

"You can't eat that!" or "What do you mean by going out and buying a bag of hmmm hmmms!" or "I saw you take that dessert when you thought nobody was looking!"

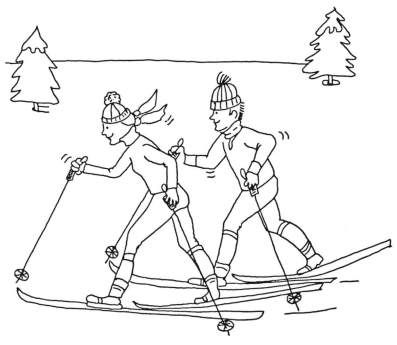

Eschewing the fat

This tough attitude of "lose weight or else . . ." never put anyone on a thinning path. In fact, it is liable to make a Sneakeater out of the most sincere would-be-thinner. Being scared into weight-losing, for fear of abandonment, may turn the dieter into a bundle of hostilities, which bodes ill both for maintaining the weight loss and the health of the relationship. Overeating becomes a crime, with the FAT-free spouse as the jailer.

The parent food warden

Ditto. A parent who becomes a drill sergeant, calling out what a child or teenager will or will not eat, just sets up a game of offspring vs. parent, overeater vs. self-proclaimed guardian of the overeater's input. A parent can help, by having the right kinds of food available, by offering non-food rewards, by encouragement and support.

But a parent cannot monitor every morsel that enters a child's mouth. In the long run, a young person has to take responsibility for his or her own body's well-being. Parent-child games get in the way of that responsibility for self.

(Note: set a firm example, to keep from passing on the FAT habit to your progeny, *Never nibble while you cook.* When your children help you put food together for a meal, make it a hard-and-fast rule that there is to be no pre-meal tasting.

"It is not necessary to eat while you cook," says a beautiful woman from Greece who concocts magnificence in her kitchen. When her young daughters aid her in culinary projects, she reports that "a Mediterranean scream" erupts at the very sight of a mixing spoon heading for a mouth, or a finger scraping a bowl en route to the same destination. "This is a principle to live by," she says. (And her family does.)

The jealous mate

The husband, wife lover who feels "ownership" may be threatened by the dieter's increasing appeal to others, now that the weight is coming off. The assumption is: A FAT

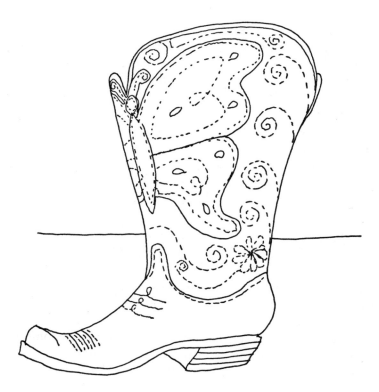

The fatted calf requires a custom boot.

wife (or husband) is a faithful one. If she (or he) is not so FAT, who knows?

Take the husband of a pretty woman who has peeled off nearly one hundred unneeded pounds. Although she has no intention of "playing around," she attracts whistles and wows for the first time in years. Doubts set him to wondering. While outwardly encouraging her, he may surprise her with sabotage — by bringing home a gallon of her once-favorite ice cream or insisting that they dine at a restaurant with no recourse for a dieter. Often the jealous mate is heedless of such dualism.

The food-bearing grandparent

This well-meaning saboteur is a product of the "food is love" school, so it is hard to blame the food-bearing grandparent, usually a grandmother. Gifts of food are ways of showing affection, winning a grandchild's approval, contributing to the younger household. She is the one who provides the foil-wrapped bunnies and gummy beans for the Easter baskets, the striped canes for the Christmas socks, the sugary shamrocks for St. Patrick's day and the Valentine heart-boxes. When she earmarks a bag of baked things for the one thin member of the house, she isn't aware of how it spreads resentment through the heavier ranks of the family. Most often, the food-bearing grandparent is a thin person.

The envious friend

This usually is a longtime friend whose life has paralleled that of the weight-loser. The relationship is well established, and competition between the two is in a balance. Now the dieter has changed all that by becoming thinner, better looking, and more self-aware — growing as a person while diminishing in scale. The friendship's long standing becomes misunderstanding, unless the non-dieting friend is honest enough to *admit* to being envious.

The in-laws who expect too much

Often this is more an exercise of the FAT person's delusions than an actuality. The heavy son-in-law is sure that he is being compared with his wife's lean father.

("He's retired. He can play golf any time he wants to. No wonder he's in shape.") The FAT daughter-in-law compares herself with her husband's trim, style-conscious mother. ("She isn't saddled with little kids. She has time for herself. I don't.") And what starts as a simple comparison of body types expands to include talents, capabilities, friendships, around-the-house skills, money-making abilities — you name it. Whatever the asset in question, the overweight in-law assumes he or she does not have it. In light of such comparisons, the heavy ones — even if they are not very heavy — feel like boobs and clods. They are not living up to what is, in their minds, expected of them as in-laws. Discouragement of this sort produces not only misery but more FAT.

The doctor who says, "Wait until you feel better before you worry about losing weight."

Does a thin doctor realize that a compulsive overeater can put on more than a few pounds while recovering from any ailment, even a short-term one? Does a medical advisor who has never struggled with too much weight know that a sweet cough syrup can send a dieter who has been off refined sugar for weeks into a binge? It is up to the weight-loser to explain that the diet plan is top priority and ask that treatment, if at all possible, be prescribed accordingly.

Are you aware of anyone who, wittingly or not, is sabotaging your weight-losing program?

How can you change yourself so that you will not be affected by such sabotage?

Parrying the praise phrase

We OWs tend to turn aside, distort and discount any and all compliments that come our way. Even if we have every right to be confident about certain aspects of our selves — our brains, our stamina, our achievements, our imagination — often we are not. The way we look, together with the lack of control that makes us look that way, maintains our self-images at snail level. Sometimes we do not even realize how consistently we deny *anything* nice that is said about us, until it is pointed out to us. Then we are amazed.

Not that we can't handle praise. We eat it up (along with a lot of food). It is just that we never quite believe it. If we are not happy with ourselves, how can anyone *else* admire us?

Do you recognize yourself here?

Thin person: "Gee, you look nice today."

Overweight: "Maybe I would if I were three sizes smaller." (Thinks: Well, you don't have to act so surprised about it!)

TP: "That color is so becoming: it matches your eyes."

OW: "My eyes are green, actually." (Thinks: You can't miss the color — there is so much of it!)

TP: "You have such a pretty face."

OW: "Flattery will get you nowhere!" (Thinks: I suppose my body is so awful that you have to concentrate on my face.)

TP: "You move so well. You must have really good coordination."

OW: "I was a dancer once — a long time ago." (Thinks: I'll bet that means "in spite of my weight.")

Consider, instead, how we put down the complimenter when we pooh-pooh the compliment. Part of learning how to care about our thin selves is to practice *accepting* compliments. Even if we detect unsaid qualifying clauses such as "in spite of your weight" or "not bad for a FAT person," we are better off ignoring them.

If we accept with grace the good things that are said about us, then the complimenter is, in turn, complimented by our acceptance. If we seem not overly sensitive about being overweight, the complimenter is likely to relax and forget about it, too.

Accepting compliments is an art — a lost art among OWs. A diet group can be a great help in pointing out to us how we parry and ward off remarks of approval.

Three cheers for me. I look nice today. I wear becoming colors. I have a pretty face. And I move well.

Thank you very much.

Can you remember any compliments you refused to accept? List them here, if you can. Don't be surprised if it is hard to remember any. We tend to strike them from our registers.

Practice giving yourself some compliments. Think of ten things you like about yourself:

1. _____
2. _____
3. _____
4. _____
5. _____
6. _____
7. _____
8. _____
9. _____
10. _____

Cultivating the thin response

Would I respond as a FAT person or as a thin person to the following situations?

1. On a walking tour of a historical neighborhood, my feet start to hurt.

2. I pass a street vendor with a wagonful of popped stuff.

3. In a game of tennis doubles, the set is 8-8 and the temperature eighty-eight degrees in the shade.

4. At an open house, doors part to reveal the glories of a magnificently laden buffet table.

5. The kitten overestimated his courage and has been sitting on the chimney for a day and a half.

FAT response	Thin response
I plop down on a park bench and let the tour go on without me.	I take off my shoes and carry them, not wanting to miss anything.
I break down and buy a bagful, even though the operation looks a little grubby.	I walk by without stopping. The operation looks a little *too* grubby for me.
I ask for a sudden-death playoff, fearing sudden death.	I request that we play it out, until one team *really* wins.
I am the first one in line, worried that the choice items may be gone if I hesitate. As I help myself, I don't mind rearranging the artistic symmetry of the platters. After all, food is to eat, isn't it? I fill my plate until it looks like a foothill of the Appalachians.	I am so busy talking with a new friend that I must be reminded to join the buffet line. I remark about the beauty of the food display, taking care to preserve it as I half-fill my plate.
I call the fire department, which refers me to the Animal Humane Society, which refers me to a private rescue team, which airlifts the kitten via pole and basket — and then collects a sizable check for the service.	I get out my extension ladder, climb it with a can of cat food and lure the kitten down.

6. A hundred or so aimless others and I are queuing up for a Saturday night movie. A brassy character elbows in and sandwiches his body between me and the person in front of me.

7. I push the "up" button in a fifteen-story office building and an almost-full elevator stops for me.

8. The following items have come to rest on the living-room floor: a rawhide dog bone, a heel-casting of dried mud, a spoon and a bowl, some toy plastic automobiles, five magazines, two cassette tapes, two tape cases, the newspaper (in sections), a cat food can which the dog lifted out of the garbage.

9. Another situation requiring folding from the waist: On a tennis court, three balls have landed widely spaced on my side of the court.

FAT response	Thin response
I sigh inaudibly and wonder to myself about the nerve of some people nowadays. I can hardly blame him, however. He probably thought I'd take up at least two seats which might keep him from getting one.	I tap him on the shoulder and say, "I'm sorry, but the end of the line is back there, a half a block away."
When I see the already crowded elevator, I turn away and pretend not to be waiting for it. I detect fear in the eyes of the passengers watching me. I can't risk not fitting, or having someone say, "Next car, please." What if I were the last straw that snapped the cables and sent it plummeting to the sub-basement?	With only a slight pause, I size up the space and, confident that there is plenty of room for me, board the elevator. Nobody blinks.
If I am a neat FAT, I harvest the mess with FAT theatrics bending, huffing and muttering about others' irresponsibility. If I am a not-so-neat FAT, I sigh and gather up the papers, while kicking the rest into one pile in the corner. I'll pick it up later in one fell swoop instead of several.	I pick them up automatically while thinking about other things. I make a mental note to deliver an ultimatum about everyone in the household picking up her/his own scatterings.
I rake and dribble them into one place with the top of my racquet — and *then* bend over to pick them up. Just one bend.	I fold over to pick up each separately. Three bends.

10. Just one small space is left on a subway bench. The persons on either side of it condense themselves as much as possible to make room and motion me to it.

11. I have settled into the next-to-the-aisle seat in a movie theater, when two latecomers say, "Excuse me," on their way to seats in the middle of my row.

12. A mouse runs across the kitchen floor.

13. I smell smoke while staying on the third floor of a small hotel. An alarm sounds.

More situations:

_____

_____

_____

_____

_____

_____

FAT response	Thin response
I shake my head no-thanks and lie, "I'd just as soon stand. I've been sitting all day." Truth is: I know I'd never fit my behind in the specified area, and it would be humiliating to not make it.	I say, "Thanks," and sit down — gratefully.
I turn my knees to one side, hoping they can crawl across me. One trips on my foot. I blush in the dark and feel terrible.	I collect my lapful of coat, get to my feet and let them pass.
I let it run over my foot as I scream operatically.	I vault up to sit calmly on the counter.
I realize that there is no way I can escape through a window via a fire department ladder. I make my way to the exit stairs — thank God, the fire is not in the stair well — and vow from henceforth to start becoming a thin person.	I don't panic. I realize that if I can't make it down the inside stairway, I can always crawl out onto the roof below and wait to be rescued. I thank God I *am* a thin person.

I respond as a FAT person:	I respond as a thin person:
_____	_____
_____	_____
_____	_____
_____	_____
_____	_____
_____	_____

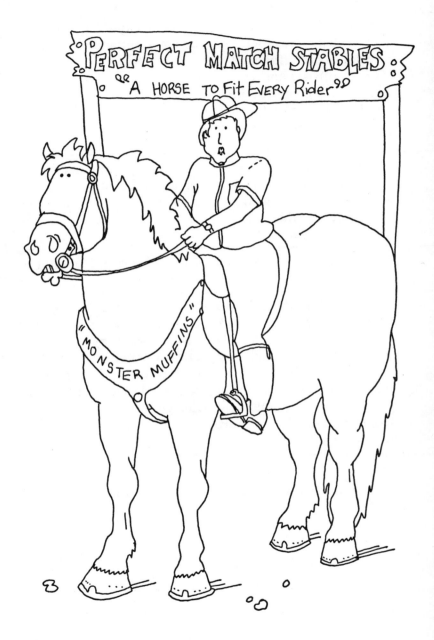

Where am I on the road to Thindom?

Check your whereabouts.

Denial of the FAT problem ("I don't like to talk about it.")
- ☐ Refusing to mention weights and measures
- ☐ Blurring eyes at the sight of self reflected in a mirror or a shop window
- ☐ Avoiding the grim truth of the scale
- ☐ Putting off shopping for clothes
- ☐ Recognizing that someone *else* might have a weight problem (but not *me!*)

Recognition of the FAT facts ("I guess I may be a little too FAT . . .")
- ☐ Making excuses for my heaviness
- ☐ Blaming
- ☐ Procrastinating about losing weight

Acceptance of the problem ("FAT is getting in my way!")
- ☐ Seriously looking at how FAT hampers my living —
- ☐ Collecting specific reasons for wanting to lose weight. Realization that help is needed ("Okay, I can't win on my own. What do I do now?")
- ☐ Exploring avenues for self-change — a group, a doctor, a daily weigh-in program, a co-losing friend, any or all of these combined with a Higher Power

Decision to make the first move ("I will pick up the phone right now!")
- ☐ Making the phone call
- ☐ Going to the meeting
- ☐ Setting up the appointment

Acquaintance with the program ("Tell me everything you can about how this works.")
- ☐ Learning the plan
- ☐ Learning about myself in relation to the plan

Pursuit of a plan ("Nothing would get me to fall away from this program now. I am really determined to do it this time!")

- ☐ Following faithfully the specified regime
- ☐ Adding appropriate exercise, other disciplines
- ☐ Finding alternatives for eating, developing new interests

Arrival at goal ("Wow! I did it!")

- ☐ Learning a maintenance food plan
- ☐ Accepting compliments with grace (but without smugness)

Maintenance of appropriate weight ("I'm thinner. I feel good. I have chosen to make the most of myself. I am beginning to be a whole person, unshackled by FAT.")

- ☐ Sticking with a maintenance food and exercise plan
- ☐ Remaining humbly wary of moments of "powerlessness"
- ☐ Leading an active, thin, lively life

Check your progress.

Fat
is not
a
moral
problem.

It's an oral problem.

Part II

Thinciples:
Listening to the thinner winners

Inner singalongs and signs,
Mottoes, props and crutches
Remind us, as they cheer us on,
Of just how much too much is.

Thinciples
How others have thinned

Why live FAT? I might never know the joys of living thin, unless I start now to work toward it. When it comes to overweight — why over-wait?

I am ready to listen to the thinner winners.

The following clues, thoughts, hints, crutches, signposts to plant inside your head come from winners at the losing battle — those who have taken off the pounds successfully. Some of these methods and techniques are sound, well-tested principles being used by diet plans and groups. Others, developed by individuals for their personal weight-losing schemes, may sound slightly kooky. The idea is: Whatever works for you, do it (if your doctor approves, of course).

We who have puffed up our normal human shapes with too much eating find our best inspiration from others like us who have *done it*, pared off said puff. What follows here is a sharing, a pooling of ideas from people who care about becoming their best thin selves — and helping other OWs to do the same.

A word first about positive thinning. Unless I think I am worth it, how can I possibly peel away the layers? This is the biggest FATtrap of all. The FATter I got, the less I thought of myself. The less I thought of myself, the FATter I got. Nothing made me feel smaller than being too big. I just knew that the thin world was fixing me with a frosty eye and muttering, "No will power," "weak," "weird," "sad," "freakish." I hid, agreeing wholeheartedly with what I imagined people were saying about me.

Here is the place to begin, the starting line:

I am worth getting thin for.

"I knew I had to make a real commitment."

Ask anyone who has taken off pounds, visibly and triumphantly, "How did you do it?" The answer begins like this: "Well, I just decided that . . . "

The rest of it may be: "I'd had enough of living this way," "I was sick and tired of being overweight," "I couldn't go on being fifty pounds heavier than my husband," "I really wanted to take up disco dancing, and imagine a FAT person bobbing around on a dance floor,"

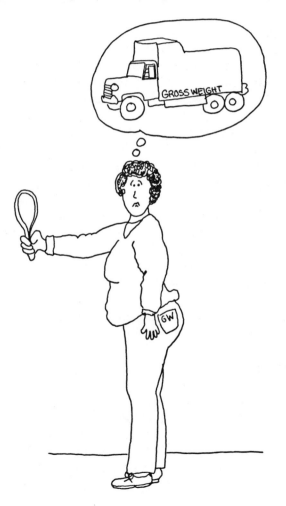

"Since I needed this operation, I *had* to lose weight," "I was running out of years to be active while I wasted them sitting in the bleachers."

The launching pad to success is those words, "I just decided that . . ."

If you need some good reasons to lose weight, list them here.

Well, I just decided that: _____

_____

_____

_____

_____

_____

_____

_____

Commitment is caring a lot at the start of the weight-losing program — and *keeping on caring*.

A weight-loser's creed:

"I believe that I can and will lose weight, steadily, surely, joyfully, until I reach my goal.

"I pray for the motivation, the inspiration, the patience and the faith to change.

"I believe that I am worthwhile, that I deserve to live life as a thin person.

"I have been given special gifts, not the least of which is life itself. I also have been given the ability to make choices. I choose to make the most of my gifts. I choose life."

Growing thinner is like looking into the lens of a camera and focusing. I adjust the outlines of my present, larger self until those lines are congruent with the outlines of the thinner self I am working toward. When the two are in focus, I will no longer be just a wishful shrinker.

"I live a day at a time."

I will not project my weight loss to next summer when I'll be back in my bikini or my golf shorts, next week when I must fit the next-size-down jeans or else, not even until the next morning's weigh-in. I know about expectations. And I know about disappointments.

I will plan my food for one day ahead, and stick to the plan. Substitutions allow room for FAT doubt: Do I really need to eat *exactly* what the diet calls for? The answer is YES.

If a day seems intolerably long, I'll try just a morning. Or just an afternoon (no late-in-the-day snacks). Or just ten minutes.

I will practice *waiting* to eat. Instead of ripping into the grocery bags en route, I will get the supplies home, fill the cupboards, put anything too tempting in the freezer, and *wait* until mealtime.

I can do without grazing — for the next five minutes, for the next half-hour, for a day at a time. I will not think about depriving myself of my love-foods "forever," or "for a year or two," just one day. Then I will deal with the following day as it comes.

I will apply the "a-day-at-a-time" principle not only to eating, but to my total pattern of living. If I have a lengthy report to finish and my thoughts are in a snarl, I will work away at it, bit by bit. If my day is tight with myriad little tasks until it seems I have no time to breathe, I will check them off, chore by chore, aiming at just those which can be finished reasonably in a day.

This is one of the most important Thinciples of all, borrowed from the philosophy of Alcoholics Anonymous and used by Twelve-Step people everywhere to help overcome compulsions of all kinds.

It works.

"I discovered that the whole answer is discipline — taking control of your life."

Get organized. Start with your purse (or your pockets). This, from an eighty-pound loser, an attractive woman in her late twenties who had existed, until a few years ago, as her parents' moon-shaped, live-in daughter. Her child-like status didn't change — nor did her shape — until she began taking over the reins to her own life, insisting on her own diet plan, pursuing her own career. Now she's riding off into the sunset confidently, unswervingly — and thinly. You would never know that she is one of us OWs. She is strict with herself, neat, beautifully groomed, creatively dressed, organized and relentlessly true to her "disciplines," which include minimal food intake pre-planned daily (no refined sugar or flour), bare shelves in her larder, inspirational daily readings, a daily walk on her noon hour, a daily hour and a half of more strenuous exercise (pick your sport), a detailed calendar of to-do's. A beautiful exception to the national statistics on post-diet recidivism, she has kept the weight off for four years.

Some simple ways to begin taking control: Keep a central calendar — just one, with *everything* on it, including what bills are due when. Remember to feed the cat on time (or you'll get your socks or your Supphose snagged). Figure out your tax in March (or earlier) instead of April. Clean your hall closet. Do your laundry before you're down to recycling your socks. Send out birthday cards in advance of the events, instead of those oops-so-sorry-I'm-late greetings. Fill the salt cellars before the salt runs out. Water your philodendron regularly, before it curtseys in an appeal for a drink.

List five ways to add discipline to your life. Write them down. Then practice doing them.

1. _____
2. _____
3. _____
4. _____
5. _____

"I do a lot of talking to myself. Even out loud."

Language. Don't underestimate it. Use it — to pep-talk yourself, to self-psych, to steer your thoughts and buttress your motivation. Whatever sort of self-talk helps — a slogan, a motto, a ditty, a jingle — say it. Tape up these sayings in key places (like the FAT's bulletin board — the refrigerator door). Borrow words from winners — from Twelve-Step programs, like Easy Does It or HALT. From self-affirming methods. (God loves me; therefore I love myself.) From anyplace — songs, hymns, poems, conversations, books, articles.

Like all compulsive people, we cling to tattered little phrases. Who cares how trite, how worn, even how silly they are. They can be effective. Whisper them. Say them out loud. Write them. Hang them up and look at them a dozen times a day. Words can be the stuff that will is built of.

Words are powerful. They can steer your thoughts to a still life of a heaping dessert — or a beach scene with you in it, decently and pleasantly thin. There I am on a beach, standing straight, not humiliated about how I look, not billowing in coverups like a circus tent being dismantled the morning after the show.

Here are some samples that have been resistance-builders for others on the thin road:

I like myself. I am worth getting thin for.

NOW is the first moment of the rest of my life.

Why weight? Don't procrastinate.

Rejoin the human race.

_____(fill in name of friend who has successfully diminished in size) did it; I can, too.

Self-control can make me whole.

Choice, not deprivation.

Pick some cheering-on words to get thin by. Let them run in your head.

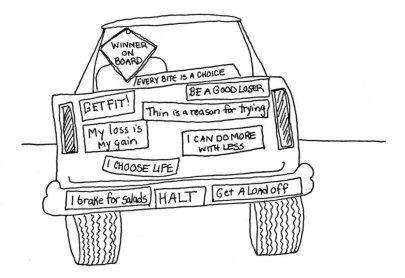

Drive your own car.

"I'm learning how to stand up for myself."

FAT is a non-assertive disease, as more and more of us are finding out. We swallow a lot of non-foods as toppings for the sundaes we used to eat — pride, for instance, and hurt, and feelings of injustice and frustration. We have to learn to look out for No. 15 (or wherever we ranked ourselves on our scale of important-to-us human beings). And one of the very first ways to be assertive is to protect our weight-losing plan from the demands of our thin fellows. "No. I plan to eat lunch at my desk today. I brought it." "No, you'll have to make your own cookies for the choir-trip sale." "I intend to spend no more than ten minutes in the kitchen. The casserole you're asking for would take me half a day to fix." When it becomes comfortable to stand firm about matters of food, try a little assertiveness in other phases of your life. It feels good.

Think of three recent instances when you stood up for yourself — and felt good about it:

1. _____

_____

_____

_____

2. _____

_____

_____

_____

3. _____

_____

_____

_____

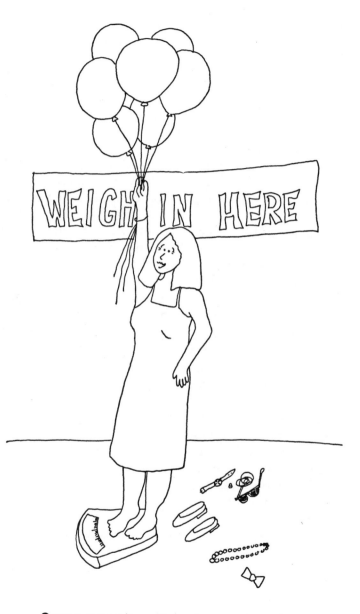

Some people will go to any lengths
to lighten up.

"I have found some new things to do that interest me, alternatives to eating."

Obviously, since food is petrol for humankind, you need it. There is no alternative to food-for-fuel. You (along with the rest of us OWs) have, however, been pumping yourself full of too rich a mixture. You need to substitute other activities. It is the eating for non-fuel reasons that plumps you — for fun, for festivity, for conviviality. You eat to live, you don't live to eat.

If you have grown up with the idea that almost nothing is more fun that eating, reconditioning is in order. No one else can tell you what *you* like to do. That requires some exploring.

A place to begin: Learn a new way of communicating — in French or Greek or Russian or German or computer language. Learn more about the world you live in, an altogether fascinating place if you are not too large and tired to notice. Take an in-depth look at a particular area of the world — or the cosmos — or a period of history that catches your fancy. Make a stab at comprehending the tensions in the Middle East. Plan a trip by jet or slow boat to China. Or simply read about it. Discover what is happening with people on the other end of the age spectrum; if you are young, take the time to meet some older folk. If you are older, tap into the energy and freshness of some young ones.

This exploration of alternative interests may require Magellan-like nerve and Columbus-like persistence. ("I am not round, even though the whole world thinks I am. Actually, I am flat.")

Try university extension classes, community classes at your local high school, outing or study clubs, neighborhood centers, YMCAs and YWCAs, art and science museums. One large downtown YWCA offered noon-hour brown-bag seminars to which you could bring your own broiled chicken and alfalfa sprouts and learn about assertiveness or economics. The lunch hour can become a learning hour, with food relegated to a minor part of it.

Though you may not believe you can squeeze a spare minute from your present schedule, you will be amazed at how much more time you have when you have lost some of your weight. It must mean that, as a heavy, you spent a lot more time eating, or preparing to eat, than you thought you did.

Name five active pursuits (sports, hobbies, projects, pastimes) that you would like to investigate:

1. _____
2. _____
3. _____
4. _____
5. _____

Discover joys of foodless places—
Motion, music, friendly faces.
Taste is one sense out of five;
Find the others. Live alive!

"I had to find my own serenity, learn to relax."

For most of us, relaxing is a learned art. It is an essential part of every weight-loss program, whether we learn it through yoga, meditation, exercise, through taking time out for ourselves to read a book or listen to music or create something beautiful, through just accepting the things we cannot change. We have to hollow out some quiet places in our lives. This may mean finding, physically, some quiet places to settle into now and then. Like these:

   in a rowboat on a pond;
   at the base of a park monument;
   on a bench in a public garden;
   on our knees in a private garden;
   on a beach warmed by sun or grayed by clouds;
   in a library carrel;
   at the back of a chapel;
   on a porch swing;
   any place but at a kitchen table or a quick-service food counter!

Your own quiet places — list them:

_____

_____

_____

_____

_____

Serenity is, of course, a state of mind. But it helps to provide yourself with a bit of quietude in your immediate environs. A reserve of serenity is needed to draw upon at times when there is a banjo twiddling bluegrass in the basement, a Spanish guitar picking classical selections in the living-room, somebody tinting her hair in the upstairs bath ("Oh, help. It turned out yellow — like the stripe on a highway!"), somebody else treating a cut foot in the kitchen, a baseball game blatting on television, a waiting automobile honking outside and some forgotten foodstuff in the oven setting off the smoke detector.

We need serenity to cope with those moments when three voices are asking simultaneous questions beginning, "Where is . . . ?"

Finding your own way to relax is a challenge. But whether it lies in newfound spiritual strength or simply preserving a small corner for your own, it is important to your well-being and your thin-being.

What have you found helpful in your pursuit of serenity?

_____

_____

_____

_____

_____

_____

_____

_____

Some methods of achieving serenity which you are willing to explore:

_____

_____

_____

_____

_____

_____

_____

_____

_____

"I learned to be aware of every bite — by staring at my food, really concentrating on it."

Zero in on your food. Give it your fully aware, undistracted, focused attention. Fix your unveering gaze upon it. Never take your eyes off your plate. Look deep into your glass or your cup. Put on your glasses if you need to. (This is preferably an at-home exercise. It will not work in a murky restaurant where you can hardly find your spoon by the flickering of a single candle.)

Think about what you are eating. Think about the concept of fueling the body by feeding it. Remember, this is why you are eating — to refuel.

What about the food? Think of how it is planted; how it sprouts in mud or sand; is chewed around the edges by other, smaller creatures; is picked, gathered, husked, culled, skinned, mashed. Or is it fattened, captured, slaughtered, reeled in, shot, sliced, ground up or deboned? Imagine the food alive, standing in a barnyard or easing through the ocean or hiding under a rock.

Observe — muster your sharpest powers of observation — how the food looks close up. Is it fibrous, grainy, wrinkled, seedy, bony, leafy, creamy, mealy, sticky? What would it feel like if it were on your fingers and not on your fork?

What do food companies do to the kinds of food you are looking at in order to can it or freeze it? Think of huge vats swimming with it.

Visualize how the food is cooked — steamed, broiled, baked, heated up.

What does it feel like in your mouth? Slippery, rough, pebbly, stemmy?

Take a half-grapefruit, for instance (an item that is acceptable on many diets and will not set us off on a food hunt).

Analyze it. Eyeball it until you can almost see the lint land on it. Each chamber, each little pouch of juice, each fat seed (some are sprouting green tendrils already), each membrane between the sections. Scrape the inside of the rind with your spoon, exposing the white inner skin. The outer skin looks almost human. Run your hand over it. Think how the fruit got that way — about big bees and citrus in the hot sun and sticky leaves and fruit hanging heavily and pickers and packers and truckers and unpackers. Think of grocery produce smells and dollars going from hand to hand and the weight of the paper bag as you carried it home. Of halving the fruit's roundness with a knife.

Describe its taste to yourself. Sweet? Not really. A slight bitterness at the back of your tongue. A sharpness on the curled tip of your tongue. How do your teeth feel? Is there a numb sensation? Does the taste stay with you?

Think of it, once scooped and used, being wrapped with the coffee grounds and eggshells, to be borne off by a noisy truck or mangled in the garbage disposer.

By the time you have traced the Life of the Grapefruit from Tree to Table (and from table to sanitation truck), you are frankly bored with the whole thing.

This little technique is not meant to be aversion therapy, which makes you think of disgusting things — like maggots — along with your favorite binge foods — a tricky process which trained bariatric professionals use only with care, if at all.

This zeroing-in process is just to make you know that you have, indeed, eaten a grapefruit. Many of us OWs eat in passing, grab as we go, so that much of the time we are unaware of what has gone into our mouths. Hence, this small lesson in realism, this exercise in awareness.

The hope is that food may lose its special allure for you and turn into plain old food, important only because it supplies nutrients to your body, but not *all*-important.

This food-awareness technique works for some. It may work for you.

"Exercise! I know I need to move — not only to help me lose weight, but for my own well-being."

Find an appropriate exercise and do it, regularly and faithfully. It is an essential part of kicking the FAT habit.

If you are unaccustomed to regular exercise, start by walking. Instead of parking your car as near as possible to your errand destinations, put a little walking distance between you and where you are going. (The great American game of automotive musical chairs is another example of greed — everybody vying for the closest parking slot to the supermarket or the restaurant or the department store.) Your body was designed to move you around, not just prop you up — give it a chance to take you at least part of the way there.

The beauty of footwork exercise is that you can build it up at your own pace — from slalk (slow walk) to walk to stride to slog (slow jog) to jog to slun (slow run) to run to sprint — adding distance as it feels right.

Check here any exercise that appeals to you and make a plan to do it. The "high" of exercise is part of the joy of thinning!

☐ judo
☐ bowling
☐ karate
☐ racquetball
☐ handball
☐ softball
   (the company team maybe)
☐ yoga
☐ tennis
☐ folk dancing

☐ interpretive dance
☐ disco dance
☐ golf
☐ basketball
☐ soccer
☐ Ping-pong
☐ hockey
☐ walking
☐ running
☐ other: _____

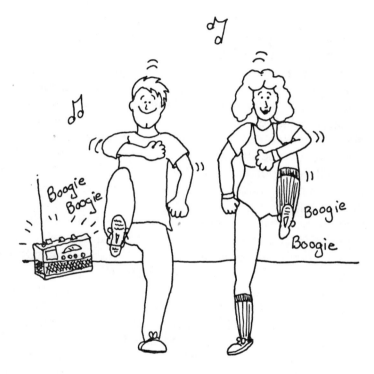

Partners in the firm

"I preview a food situation — dress-rehearse it — so that I can cope with it successfully when it happens."

This is the preview that avoids the déjà vu. (Drat it! I did it again — gave in to the same old temptation. It seems to me I've seen this scene before.) Stiff-arm temptation with this technique. Look ahead. Set the scene exactly as you foresee that it will be.

The room. Candlelit. Cushiony, but formal. The people — a bunch of pencil-like friends, making luring remarks like, "Oh, come on. There's hardly any sugar in it," or, "After all, this comes only once a year. You have to celebrate!" The music — lulling, don't care music. The conversation — centering on the world economy, comparative religions or some other subject of vast consequence guaranteed to demote your personal priority (thinning yourself) to somewhere much lower on your list of what is important. The food — works of art, loaded with gourmet sauces and sugary glazes. How will you deal with it?

Stake out your priorities before you get there. What is topmost in *your* considerations? Finding a thin self. Hang perspective! Dare to be selfish! Sometimes you have to be narrow-minded to become narrow-bodied.

Zelda is slipping a dessert plate in front of you. No-thank-you-Zelda to the plate. (If you take the plate, you will be tempted to fill it with whatever is passed next.) Too late. Pick up the plate and give it to the person next to you. Never mind manners. This is survival, not savoir-faire. Whew. Of course, you will have your regrets, when you see whatever wondrous, shimmering, towering chef d'ouvre you are denying yourself. But you have blockaded a possible slip. And tomorrow you will feel marvelous.

Now, run through the scene again, down to the last detail — even to the design on Zelda's dessert plates.

Preview your temptations, and practice your reactions. By the time the real situation comes along, your "no,

FAT myth;

A FAT person eats a lot of many different kinds of food.

FAT truth:

A FAT person usually eats few kinds of foods — but those in large quantities.*

---

*Jurgen M. Wolff and Dewey Lipe, Ph.D., *Help for the Overweight Child, A Parent's Guide to Helping Children Lose Weight* (New York: Stein and Day, 1978).

thank you" will be automatic. How can you perfect your no's unless you rehearse and rehearse and dress-rehearse them?

Set up a sample food situation for yourself here — a dinner out at a restaurant, a supper among friends, a family reunion picnic, a client luncheon, a swing through the drive-in, a wedding reception. Take yourself through it step by step. Do away with any suddenly seductive food situations by being ready for them.

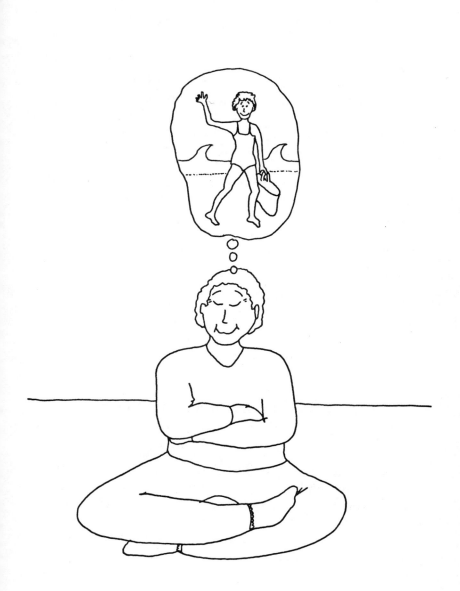

Visualize yourself thin—and smiling

"I stay away from crash, get-thin-quick regimes."

Let the faddists and the experimenters and the happy hunchers explore these. Have those who wired their jaws shut or who lived with pressure above the upper lip been able to experience the joy of thinning? Have the crash-dieters learned anything about long-term stay-thin eating, about adequate eating instead of overeating as a way of life?

This book is about triumph and accomplishment and changing lifetime attitudes for the healthier — not about deprivation.

"I plan my food a day ahead and stick with the plan."

(See sample daily chart on page 278.)

Check here when you have kept your chart for one week:_____

Check here when you have kept your chart for one month: _____

"Whenever I am starved and about to tear into a meal, I drink a glass of water first."

This is another good way to help fill your inner hollows with non-calories. Actually, they are not hollows at all. Try not to think of your "emptiness," your "hunger," your "hollowness." Let your mind dwell upon your limbs instead of your central interior. Think of the muscles tightening in your legs and arms as you add to your program of exercise — and how good that new-found muscular strength and efficiency feels. Then think of the why-did-I-eat-all-THAT discomfort that follows self-stuffing. The firm-muscle feeling wins every time!

"Slow down your eating. I was a gulper and a bolter who could put away twice as much food in the space of a suppertime as a normal eater."

Some suggestions on how to cut down your eating acceleration: Wait for a specified number of seconds to elapse between bites; put down your fork or spoon between bites; chew thoroughly. Let each bite be just that — a bite — instead of a mouthful. Eat with chopsticks — guaranteed to slow you down unless you are skilled in this traditional Far Eastern custom.

"I put a padlock on the kitchen."

Yes, someone we know really did this.

Or open up the kitchen for a brief time just before meals — as most college fraternities do, in order to keep Attaturk and his hordes from ravaging the pantry. In today's houses and apartments, where dividers have replaced walls with doors, where "areas" have replaced rooms, this lock-up-the-food trick is not always possible. What *is* possible is to give the house or apartment a new focus point — a new, appealing, comfortable gathering place — *outside* the kitchen. Step No. 1: As we said before, remove the television from the kitchen.

What specifically can you do to change the focus of where you live to another room, away from the food preparation center:

_____

_____

_____

_____

_____

_____

_____

_____

"I set up a system of rewards for myself."

Try not to establish a distant, looming, fantastic reward at the end of a monumental weight loss — a trip around the world after one hundred pounds are gone, or a new BMW or Honda (now that you are small enough to fit in one) after you have taken off fifty. Such mighty rewards may provide impetus for some. But a series of smaller rewards may be just as effective — a new shirt or blouse after the first five, a new pair of slacks after ten, a new swimsuit, a weekend vacation, a bicycle, a book, a membership in a neighboring Melting Pot (a spa or health club or park board exercise class), a series of tennis lessons. Make the reward fit the accomplishment — let it match your new, active, thin style of living.

Reasonable rewards especially for you:

At five pounds off, I deserve a _____

At ten off, I will give myself a _____

At fifteen, _____

At thirty, _____

"I use my bones as checkpoints — how they look and especially how they feel."

Bones are useful gauges. When the weight begins to vanish, the bones start to emerge from their fleshy cushions. Feel your shoulder region. The feel (or non-feel) of these bones can tell you better than a scale or a mirror what your progress has been. When you can catch rain in your clavicle, then you will know you have done it!

About hidden shoulder blades and kneecaps

Each Hershey, Heath, or Whitman Sampler
That we allowed the world to sell us
Has helped obscure, as we grew ampler,
Our scapulas and our patellas.

"I picked up some of those mirrored tiles at Sears and stuck them on the door of the refrigerator."

"Then I could *see* the compulsive gleam in my eye — greed written all over my face — when I headed for a snack." The principle behind it: When you can actually see it, your own greed makes you stop and think. Variations on the watch-yourself-about-to-binge ideas are:

1. Watch yourself chewing. Sit in front of a mirror and view your own masticatory motions, the vigorous action of your jaw hinges, the rubbery mouth movements. How long does it take to bore you out of your mind? To bring on a scream, an ugh or a yuk?
2. Watch another OW chewing. There you are, reflected in the behavior of someone very much like you. Imagine that person watching *you* chew. What do you see? What does that big chewer see in *you?*

"When in doubt, spit it out."

Not pretty. But safe. If you are abstaining from sugar and find yourself with a sweet something on your tongue — whether you put it there voluntarily or thoughtlessly — get rid of it before it becomes part of you.

"When I feel a pang of unreasonable hunger, I take a bath."

Some call this hydrotherapy. In plain fact, it is a good old peaceful soak in a tub. Half-sunken and water-soothed, you sometimes are able to switch off your appetite, maybe because eating and submerging usually are not linked activities. When you grow thinner, you will notice triumphantly that your body has pulled away from the sides of the tub; the moat around the bloat has widened!

"I have made the scale my best friend. I weigh in regularly."

Don't waste time; step on it (the scale). In spite of those who tell you not to weigh every day, thousands are peeling off FAT layers by monitoring their losses on a daily basis. Weekly weigh-ins are fine for some. For others, they are just not enough. (If you are on a weekly weighing program, do you send up a sigh of relief after each week's tally, then promptly relax your eating habits until two days before the next weigh-in?)

During those rocky moments when you knew you were gaining weight, did you — like so many of the rest of us OWs —steer clear of the scale altogether? Make elaborate excuses not to step on it ("Oh, I don't have a scale anymore; I let a friend borrow it" or "My scale is just not working right; it must be broken")? Did your rocky moments turn into rocky weeks or half-years before desperation caught up with you? Then remember the moment when you, prepared for horror, set your jaw and climbed gingerly upon it?

One hundred-pound winner drove five miles every weekday to her doctor's office without fail until the weight came off. Several programs are based on similar, never-falter systems involving daily weigh-ins. Others ask for a weight check three times a week. (Of course, if you are in a program that meets weekly, you can always develop the discipline of daily-come-what-may weigh-ins at home.)

If you care a lot about minor vacillations in your weight, wear the same clothes every day for your weigh-in. (Make that nylon parachute fabric!) One woman we know wore the same dress every day for six months; after stepping on the scale she'd race back home and change for the rest of her day.

The scale is the greatest of all confronters. Let it be your ally.

FAT and its after-math

It is not πr^2
It is $I r^2$
From eating too much π

When a minus is a plus

From the neck to the chin, my angle
Is now acutely less obtuse.
For I now fit in a thin triangle
With a short hypotenuse.

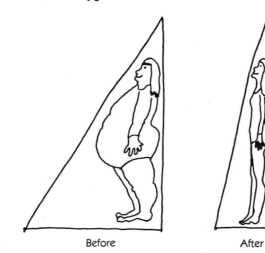

Before   After

"I have a dog with a large appetite. I share my food."

This says it.

Hungry Doggerel

Get in shape for a game of leapfrog:
Share your crumbs with your Shetland Sheepdog.

Hope to sun outside your yard? Then
Throw your scraps in your St. Bernard pen.

Want to regain a useful lap? So
Give what's left to your Lhaso Apso.

So's to reduce the size of your assets:
Offer your tidbits to your Bassetts.

Wish you had less leg than trouser?
Give your seconds to your Schnauzer.

This time, if you aim to zip it,
Save leftovers for your Whippet

Sick and tired of your nickname, "Oodles"?
Scrape your plate for your pair of Poodles.

In essence:

Beneath each table where you may dine —
Post a hungry, begging canine!

(But be sure you are not shorting your handy little four-legged garbage disposers on nutrition, or overfattening them as you trim yourself.)

"I rearrange my schedule — juggle events in my day to keep me away from food at times when I may be hungry or anxious."

If you are the chief cook in your house, plan to prepare the necessary meals at hours when you are *not* hungry and *not* anxious. Get supper ready in the morning, so that it requires just a last-minute warm-up. If you must entertain with food, get it organized well ahead of time, and steer clear of the otherwise inevitable rushing around and pre-tasting. Learn the art of make now, bake later.

An OW who is subject to numerous dinner invitations wards off overconsumption at these occasions by eating early, in the late afternoon.

How can you scramble your schedule to remove yourself from food temptations at moments when you feel your resistance may be low?

_____

_____

_____

_____

_____

_____

_____

_____

_____

_____

_____

_____

_____

"I make the pounds off really mean something by setting reasonable goals for myself."

Just seeing that needle going down on the scale is a joy in itself. But, to keep our motivation up while the number of pounds goes down, some of us need more than that. We need to keep telling ourselves *why* we are going gung-ho, full tilt, great guns at our weight-losing project. Let's translate pounds off into just what those losses mean for us: paring down in time for a vacation; lowering blood pressure; reducing life insurance premiums; joining the Gymtown Joggers without fear of overtaxing a big body; easing into a pair of shorts by the Fourth of July picnic.

Five pounds off is not just five pounds off. It is making the team. It is a half-size smaller. It is a new buckle hole in your belt or a compliment from an old friend. Keep it simple — and reasonable. Turn pounds lost into something else gained. And plug away at your losing, a day at a time.

What is the most important meaning of your pounds off?

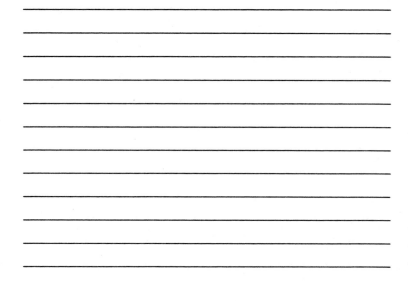

"I keep a Mother Hubbard cupboard — bare."

If other members of the household want crackling snacks or sweet crisps around, let them keep such evils (for you) out of your sight. Strip your immediate environment — at home or at work — of foods that lure. (Are you substituting another binge food — something that had not tempted you heretofore — for one that you have carefully erased from your life? A common FATfall for those who have "housecleaned.")

Check here if you have cleaned up your food environment: ☐

"Whenever I feel my priorities about to shift, I concentrate on 'better than's.' "

Like these:

Moving lightly is better than a frozen-bar-on-a-stick.

Good health is better than stuffy satiety.

Control is better than eat-everything chaos.

A bag lunch that follows my diet plan is better than a devil-may-care splurge at lunch time that I will regret for the rest of the day.

Feeling good about myself is better than three minutes' worth of tasting something sweet.

A la thin is better than à la mode.

A fresh salad is better than a pudding-filled pastry.

Freedom is better than slavery to foods.

Add your "better than's" here:

_____

_____

_____

_____

_____

_____

Which way will you go when you come to the fork in the road?

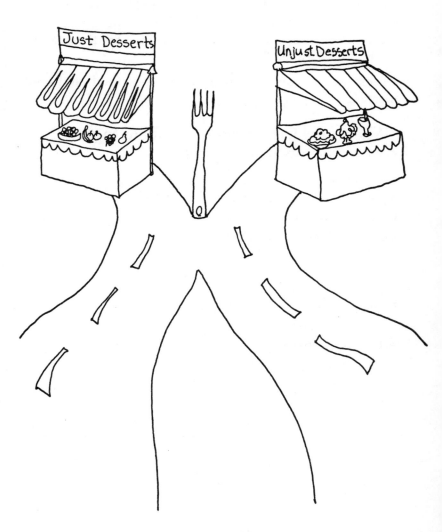

Will you choose Just Desserts?
Or Unjust Desserts?

Just Desserts
Melon balls
Sliced peaches
Apples cooked without
  sugar
Fresh strawberries
Fresh raspberries
Fresh blueberries
Air pudding
Illusion
An orange
A half-grapefruit

Unjust Desserts
Torte Huge
Gooey Louis
Creme de la Creme
Frappe Trap
Whippeau d'Elephant
Gateau soaked in Grog de
  Magog
Whippety Doodah
La Mousse Grosse
Une Bombe
White Mountain Meringue
  (Mont Blanc)

Hints on the eve of your decision:
A torte distorts. A meringue makes you overhang. A
mousse turns you into one.

"I eat only from small dishes."

Put away those vast, buffet-sized dinner plates. Use salad plates, or even saucers, upon which a dab of food looks like a feastly heap. One woman reported borrowing her four-year-old's doll plates. She said it cut down her intake noticeably.

"I never serve food from platters anymore."

Remove your option to take seconds. Fill your plate once, with exactly what you need to eat. Don't give yourself the chance for "just a little more" — and a little more — and a little more — and why not clean it up?

"I never grocery-shop on an empty stomach."

Shop after you have eaten. Shop from a list and stick to it. Be brisk and business-like about it. Don't loiter. Skip the aisles where temptation lurks.

If you are avoiding sugar, read the lists of ingredients on the food packages. You may be surprised to find that it is among the first mentioned ingredients. Are you being slipped the sweets when you are not even aware of it?

Anti-temptation strategy

If you buy a treat as a family-pleaser,
Tuck it safely in the freezer.
For a frozen goodie sticks in your craw,
Chips your molar or breaks your jaw.
And by the time you've let it sit and thaw —

      You've forgotten about it.

"I have learned to wrap all the leftovers in foil or put them in containers I can't see through."

Same principle as the above.

Qualifier: If you are one who can't stand the sight of a mystery package without undoing its wrappings, this handy-hint probably won't do a thing for you.

"If I eat something I know I shouldn't — or if I want to tone down a desire to eat — I rinse my mouth with mouthwash."

An overwhelmingly, eye-wateringly minty (or whatever) mouthwash can preempt all taste-images of food. Gum (the sugarless kind) can have the same effect of erasing a food-longing, besides keeping the mouth busy and out of trouble, which brings us to a related point:

"I am not a bit shy anymore about asking for a People Bag at a restaurant."

When eating out, you don't have to consume on the spot every last morsel served up to you just because you're paying for it. Take home the leftovers. Spread out the feast over a couple of days. You'll save your funds and your figure.

"I found that I had to discover what my eating cues were — and then remove them."

What are your cues to eat? A time of day? An event? A certain setting — a table or a counter or a specific kind of dinnerware? Even a rose pattern on a dessert plate can turn you on if you are accustomed to seeing that rose next to a baked marvel. The *Laugh It Off* daily chart on page 278 may help you discover what some of these cues are. Do away with them. Or substitute non-cues. For example, a simple oriental plate that brings to mind beautifully prepared vegetables instead of that rose-patterned dessert plate that has added too much romance to your gloppy-sweets eating.

Others have professed to salivate at the sound of a telephone ringing in the kitchen, at the sight of a food ad on television, at the crinkle of a paper bag, at a food smell emanating from the oven, at the sizzle of a barbecue on the balcony of a neighboring apartment.

Another successful dieter came up with this corollary:

"In order to quit giving myself cues to eat, I stopped referring to meals as 'breakfast,' 'lunch,' 'supper,' 'dinner.' I just call them loosely: morning food (or noon or evening food)."

Far-fetched? Maybe. Only you can identify the cues that switch on the appetite. And only you can think of turn-off methods.

Your cues: **How to avoid them:**

_____   _____

_____   _____

_____   _____

_____   _____

_____   _____

_____   _____

And a few more:

"Someone in my diet group told me to take the bulb out of the refrigerator."

You will be amazed at how dingy and gray food scraps look unlighted. You'll find it considerably harder to cue yourself to eat when you can't see what you're after. Just imagine, as an example, the difference between a full-color food ad and one in black and white.

"I make sure I have plenty of things to do that can't be combined with eating. And I do them."

You cannot eat and do any of the following:
chew gum;
chase a fly with a swatter;
drink water at a fountain;
brush your teeth;
kiss;
swim underwater (just being in cold water uses up extra calories);
plant;
give a talk;
perform an appendectomy;
teach a class;
sing;
whistle;
hang clothes on a line (you need your mouth as a clothespin holder);
thread a needle;
pilot a boat in a windstorm;
take your temperature;
dictate a letter;
lick an envelope;
refinish a floor;
run.

What else? _____

_____

_____

_____

_____

_____

_____

_____

"I make sure I get plenty of sleep. I have trouble dieting when I am really tired."

If you are a night person who is inclined to prowl and putz around your dwelling-place after most of the world is asleep, you may be overeating to make up for lack of sleep. Analyze your sleep habits. Make it easier on yourself. Don't count on energy from food as a substitute for the renewal that comes from a decent night's sleep.

And, in general . . .

Don't bite off more than you can chew.
Don't chew more than you should swallow.
Don't swallow more than you need to live
as a healthy, thin person.

The preceding list of Thinciples which have helped other OWs along their way comprises only a smattering of successful methods for change. The next pages provide room to add your own discoveries.

Your own Thinciples may be as profound and soul-shaking as discovering a new spiritual path or as frivolous as tacking a poster of Cheryl Tiegs on your refrigerator or taping cartoons of pigs on your cupboards (depending on whether you respond to positive or negative reminders).

Your own Thinciples here:

_____

_____

_____

_____

_____

_____

_____

_____

_____

_____

_____

_____

_____

_____

_____

_____

_____

_____

_____

_____

_____

_____

Your own Thinciples:

_____

_____

_____

_____

_____

_____

_____

_____

_____

_____

_____

_____

_____

_____

_____

_____

_____

_____

_____

_____

_____

_____

_____

_____

_____

_____

_____

Part III

The Thindown: Doing it

When I try to change the things I can,
Don't wish me luck, but a plan.
When I vow no more to overfill,
Don't wish me luck, wish me will.
When I choose to lose to stay alive,
Don't wish me luck, wish me drive.
When I turnabout from observer to player,
It's not luck I need — it's your prayer.

Countdown for the Thindown
(from one to thirty)

I have appraised the size of my body. My considered opinion: too big.

I have looked at myself statistically, in the honest light of reality, in a mirror *not* steamed up from the shower which makes me look like a cumulus cloud at sunset, in a shop window *not* plastered with special sale posters. Now that I have stripped off a few defenses, bared a few flimsy excuses, exposed some FAT fantasies that stand in the way of success — I'm ready — Lord, am I ready — to unload some unwanted weight.

I am now ready to stop blaming, excusing, procrastinating, hemming, hawing and pretending it isn't there. I am entirely aware of the differences between living a full life thin and a less full life FAT. I know what I am missing. I am not going to settle for missing it any longer.

I am also aware, after years of creeping upwards weight-wise that I need help — from others who have won at losing, and from God.

Like the alcoholic, I, as a compulsive overeater, do not have to wait for a moment of truth — a doctor's decree, a friend's confrontation, a mate's "I really wish you were thinner." I can gear up to thin down any time. **NOW.**

Nobody notices anything yet: but you know there has been a momentous, glorious change — you have finally, at long last, decided to find your thin self under all those puffy pounds.

No more charting pounds off on a daily graph. Every weight-loss chart I have tried to keep has ended up looking like ricrac or the dorsal fin on a stegosaurus. This time I will try something different.

Each two-page spread from this point on until the end of this book will represent one pound. I will turn the page and go on to the next only after losing the pound in question.

In other words, this will be a sort of FAT Pilgrim's Progress, recorded humbly and gratefully, in the hope that any insights and discoveries along the way will have some meaning for other chubs on the same joyful journey.

The theory is: If I — a chronic dieter, a multifold repeater, can do it — anybody can!

And if I wake up some shining morning and can turn two pages for a two-pound loss — huzzah! Double hooray for me!

If I am set back a pound and have to flip a page the other way, at least my temporary gain is not recorded as an unalterable, discouraging mountain peak in the rugged topography of my weight-losing terrain. I invite my will-be-thinner readers to do the same — turn a page per pound. Are you with me, fellow FATS?

I have chosen thirty pounds as a round number to lose on our way to becoming less round. Some of us will find our thin selves sooner, at five off, or seven, or fifteen or twenty-seven and a half. If so, stay with us until you've lost your prescribed number, then skim the rest. If you have (as I have) more than thirty extra, carry on in the same style. Flip the pages. Happy flipping.

Here you are, a mighty challenge to yourself. Begin right now to imagine yourself as a thinner person, doing thinner things. You have a long row to hoe, but at least by the end of it you'll be able to bend over to do it! Get fired with the excitement of CHANGE. FAT is a progressive disease.

Now is the time for all good overweights to come to the aid of their bodies.
Now is the time for all good overweights to come to the aid of their bodies.
Now is the time for all good overweights to come to the aid of their bodies.
Now is the time for all good overweights to come to the aid of their bodies.
Now is the time for all good overweights to come to the aid of their bodies.
Now is the time for all good overweights to come to the aid of their bodies.
Now is the time for all good overweights to come to the aid of their bodies.
Now is the time for all good overweights to come to the aid of their bodies.
Now is the time for all good overweights to come to the aid of their bodies.
Now is the time for all good overweights to come to the aid of their bodies.
Now is the time for all good overweights to come to the aid of their bodies.
Now is the time for all good overweights to come to the aid of their bodies.
Now is the time for all good overweights to come to the aid of their bodies.
Now is the time for all good overweights to come to the aid of their bodies

and their minds and their spirits and their self-images and their
creativity and their productivity and their abilities to love
and their capacities for fun and their propensities for good
relationships and their feelings of general well-being.

Yes. NOW IS THE TIME.

You feel an inkling — just an inkling — of tentative happiness.

Equivalent: One medium-sized acorn squash.

Finally, after a couple of false starts and a holiday snag, the first pound has melted off. I tripped over St. Valentine's commemorative love-is-food festivities getting here. A teenage friend brought me a heart-shaped baked offering, and I was so touched that I ate a piece — and put off the losing until the next day. If this sounds like a copout — it was, but hopefully one that occurs only *before* an actual trimdown begins. (See FATfalls, No. 1.)

I know that I will have to find new, non-gastronomical methods of coping with the family activities jam which takes place regularly between the hours of 4 and 6 p.m. Some sample pre-dinner scenes from my house:

Daughter needs poster board for school speech project. NOW! Otherwise she will fail speech class. Heaven forbid. Rush to a dimestore to pick up posterboard. Sail like a schooner through parking lot as wind catches posterboard under arm. Return to find dangling phone receiver, with neighbor woman on end of the line. Our adolescent tomcat is maowing on her doorstep. What does she expect when she has a female cat still in business? Apologize to neighbor, nice as pie. (Oops. There I go with a food image. Nice as a spring day. Nice as velvet. Nice as anything but pie.) Say, sweetly, "I just hadn't realized that our cat was old enough to care. He must be precocious." Think, less sweetly, "Whose problem is it, anyway?" Retrieve little tomcat and call vet for appointment to remedy the situation. (Why doesn't *she* call *her* vet?) Open refrigerator door. "No," to self. Close it. Phone goes *brr-r-r-r-ing*. Get out the vote for mayor. *Brr-r-r-r-ing* again. Where is overdue collection envelope currently circulating around neighborhood. Promise to track it down. Dog is roaring at newspaper carrier. Since carrier is smaller than dog, hide dog, still roaring, in back bedroom. *Brr-r-r-r-ing* twice. "No, she's not here; she's at choir rehearsal. Yes, I'll leave a note that it's REALLY IMPORTANT for her to call you." *Brr-r-r-r-ing.* "No, he's not." (Oh-oh, it's a client, and I sound grumpy as a troll under a bridge. Try to soften the grump with a lighter, more receptive tone.) "He is still at the office. Would you like to call him there? I'm sure he would be happy to hear from you." I catch myself eating ruffles of salad greens, phone receiver clamped between chin and shoulder, while trying to throw something together for supper. There. See? My response to everyday chaos is absolutely predictable: Feed the face. This emphasizes my long-held theory of Chub from Hubbub. It is not hunger that drives me to eat. It is frazzled nerves. It is disorganization. It is reacting to crises instead of planning ahead to avoid them. A few changes are in order.

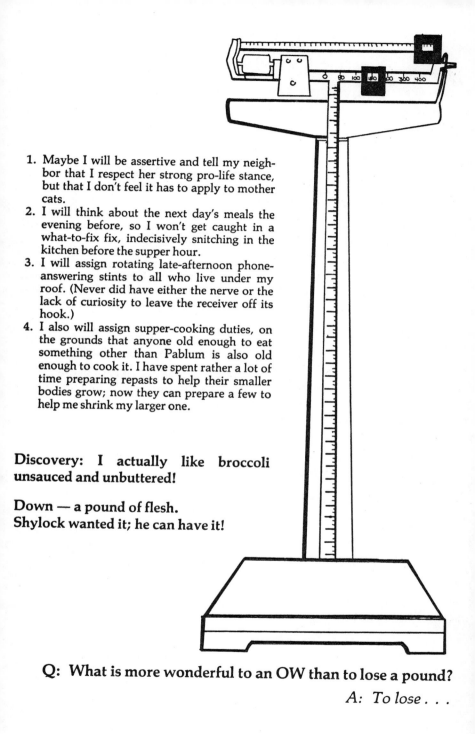

1. Maybe I will be assertive and tell my neighbor that I respect her strong pro-life stance, but that I don't feel it has to apply to mother cats.
2. I will think about the next day's meals the evening before, so I won't get caught in a what-to-fix fix, indecisively snitching in the kitchen before the supper hour.
3. I will assign rotating late-afternoon phone-answering stints to all who live under my roof. (Never did have either the nerve or the lack of curiosity to leave the receiver off its hook.)
4. I also will assign supper-cooking duties, on the grounds that anyone old enough to eat something other than Pablum is also old enough to cook it. I have spent rather a lot of time preparing repasts to help their smaller bodies grow; now they can prepare a few to help me shrink my larger one.

Discovery: I actually like broccoli unsauced and unbuttered!

Down — a pound of flesh. Shylock wanted it; he can have it!

Q: What is more wonderful to an OW than to lose a pound?

A: To lose . . .

Your mother notices.

Equivalent: Two pounds of butter. Imagine them tied to your belt, one over each hip.

I'm learning to start my day the evening before — with a plan of *exactly* what kind of food and how much of it I will put into myself during the following day. I won't just speculate about my food plan. I'll write it down, stare at it and plot how to implement it. That way I won't get caught with my resistance down, happily pouncing on excuses to procrastinate, like these:

The no-wheels-no-deal excuse. Oh-oh. Imagine my stupidity! Dummy — that's me! — forgot to pick up a can of water-packed tuna. Guess I'll have to whip over to the supermarket and get one. Oh-oh again. I told Zeb he could take the car to the council meeting. Too bad. I'll just have to settle for fish swimming in oil — and the attendant calories.

Or the old cold-turkey ploy. "Gee, I should have taken that bird out of the freezer sooner. It will never thaw in time to roast it for supper. How about something from the corner Duke Burger instead?"

Even more effective than just writing down what I'm going to eat the following day, is to read the plan over the phone to an also-thinning friend first thing in the morning.

. . . Get Set, Go!

What — precisely what — will launch me
On my way to being paunch-free?
Just the choice of what to swallow.
Just a plan that I can follow.
Just the caring to pursue it.
Just the faith that I CAN DO IT . . .

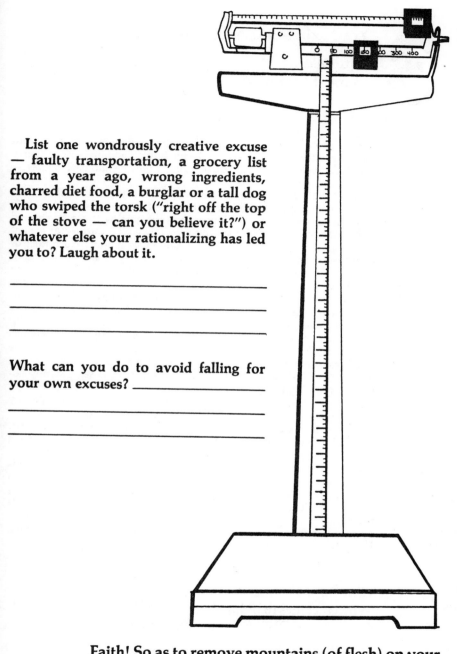

List one wondrously creative excuse — faulty transportation, a grocery list from a year ago, wrong ingredients, charred diet food, a burglar or a tall dog who swiped the torsk ("right off the top of the stove — can you believe it?") or whatever else your rationalizing has led you to? Laugh about it.

_____

_____

_____

What can you do to avoid falling for your own excuses? _____

_____

_____

Faith! So as to remove mountains (of flesh) on your way to . . .

Your skin is loosening up.

Equivalent: Three one-pound packages of meat loaf mixture.

If this process of growing smaller seems slow-as-forever, I will remember how long it took to make me into a pudding-person. Thirty years? Ten years? Six, four, three years? Rome — and FAT bodies — were not built in a day.

Here's one for the bariatric scientists. What is the ratio of the time it takes to gain, say, ten pounds, to the time it takes to lose it? While the losing always *seems* to take longer than the gaining, I can be cheered on by the histories of ex-FATs who have taken off a thirty-year weight gain in a single year, or a three-year gain in six months. Such tales of success seem to point to a happy thought, namely, that if I am loyal to my commitment, my more-than-necessary flesh will melt in less time than it took to build it up. Especially since I have been heretofore the original Marjorie Daw on her seesaw of gain-and-lose-and-gain again.

I don't feel starved. I don't feel deprived. In fact, I am elated with my progress. Then why do I seem just a little edgy? Do I sense a slight rankling, a restlessness? Am I at last unblanketing some food-tranquilized feelings? Could it be that, in spite of all my self-talk and the solidness of my resolution, I feel left out of the whole, carefree eating world? Do I feel sorry for my oversized self when I see a skinny co-worker grinning over a bake-shop splurge? Or when a much thinner member of my family engages in ambulatory munching right under my plump nose? Never before have I resented munch noises — certainly not my own. I find that the only answer, for now, is to remove myself, physically and mentally, from the petty annoyance of watching someone else consume something that I know is not good for ME.

Only "positive thinning" works for me. Not: I *won't* indulge in foods that add to my weight burden, which sets up an inner battleground between should's and shouldn't's and wears me out. Instead: I *choose* to be a healthy, thin person, and will therefore eat only what is necessary to live thin. My thinning is a positive process through which I aim to explore my joyful possibilities as an active, creative, spiritual being. So who's deprived?

When it comes to living thin, not FATter,
It's not the DON'T'S but the DO'S that matter.

220

Write here a couple of Do's that work
best for you: _____

_____

_____

_____

_____

_____

_____

_____

_____

_____

Laugh it off. Let it go.
Three down. Twenty-seven to go.

You are entirely ready for a minus . . .

221

Your roommate notices.
Equivalent: Eight solid Idaho baking potatoes.

Aha. I just dropped into a brand-new "decade" — below one of those ten-pound markers (220, 190, 180, 170, 160, 140 or whatever) that seem to hook you, keep you there, squirming and stuck, much longer than any of the in-between pound readings. Maybe if we had been brought up on metrics, we wouldn't run into these psychological snags at the ten-pound marks. I worked free of this one, floated on by it, and am now heading downward again.

Some images to play around with: I have been pinned in inactivity in a one-person spacecraft, drifting through blue-gray unreality and nothingness. Now, at last, I am headed back toward earth — where the music is, where people laugh and work and accomplish and dance and move around. With every pound lost, I am closer to rejoining the human community. I am Dorothy going home to Kansas. Now that the real world is becoming more inviting, I am chucking my fantasies along with my pounds. Thin is home. And there is no place like it!

The thin within

Can't you see that I am a dancer?
Can't you tell by the way I move?
Underneath this quilted flesh,
This pain of mass tugged down
By gravity, there is a slighter,
Nimbler form —
Beetle-quick,
Alert to tempos,
Spare as necessity
Made to translate
Joyful noise to motion.
Can't you see that I am a dancer?
Behind this self-obscuring,
Plush,
Stage-heavy
Curtain?
Can't you tell by the way I move?

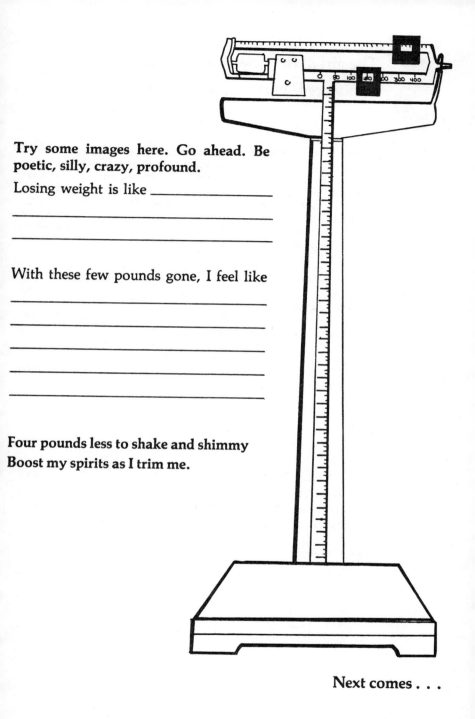

Try some images here. Go ahead. Be poetic, silly, crazy, profound.

Losing weight is like _____

_____

_____

With these few pounds gone, I feel like

_____

_____

_____

_____

_____

Four pounds less to shake and shimmy
Boost my spirits as I trim me.

Next comes . . .

The girl at the desk next to you notices.
Equivalent: Forty tennis balls.

Now here I am at the exact weight I tallied on the eve of my son's birth. I have passed by this particular mark several times since — coming and going. Funny, how different the same reading on the scale looks on the way up and on the way down. What a difference the trend makes! The identical reckoning that once stirred up tears of despair now brings a feeling of elation! Imagine the change in perspective that has me hopping for joy when I weigh exactly what I did at nine-and-a-half months pregnant. And that was a watermelon weight which all hung in one place. Now it is pasted all over me.

Nevertheless, the direction is down, down, down.

Although it is too soon for the world to note any major alteration in my appearance, I, for one, detect a certain shrinkage in the midriff area. The Michelins are deflating. Besides the daily weigh-in, I have added an everyday schedule of exercise — ten sit-ups on a padded, angled board, performed at the same time each morning, before I attack the day's hurlyburly. The routine of it seems to be as important as the exercise itself because it helps establish a mood of control, of *choosing* what I will do with my day, instead of letting the day's activities choose ME.

An exercise in memory — to test how long you have worried about your weight: When did you last pass by this particular weight (whatever you weigh now that you have lost five pounds)?

_____

_____

_____

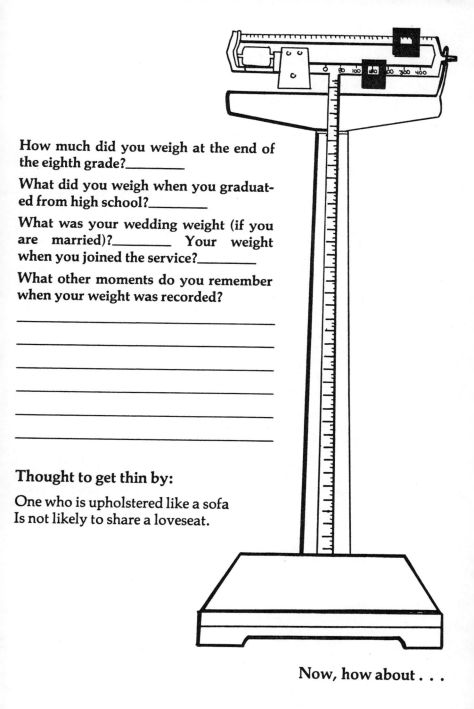

How much did you weigh at the end of the eighth grade?_____

What did you weigh when you graduated from high school?_____

What was your wedding weight (if you are married)?_____ Your weight when you joined the service?_____

What other moments do you remember when your weight was recorded?

_____

_____

_____

_____

_____

_____

Thought to get thin by:

One who is upholstered like a sofa
Is not likely to share a loveseat.

Now, how about . . .

Your shoes are loose.

Equivalent: One slow-burning fireplace log that lasts for three hours.

Past the familiar five, my old dieting ground — those first few often-lost-often-gained-back pounds. On to six now, and to territory I have not seen for a while. More and more, I am discovering that discipline and routine are essential to my successful losing, as they are for several other FATfighters I have known. Meals at regular times, for instance. No more haphazard slapped-together suppers at 11 p.m. No more "Hmmmm, what'll I have to eat?" which results in a little of this, a little of that, adding up to a lot of both.

Now that I have chosen a path to travel, I will stick with it instead of doing my usual diet-hopping. I have bounced from Atkins to eggs-and-grapefruit to elixir of seaweed to liquid protein to Scarsdale to the "I can do it my way" method. Never one to approach any diet without adding my own dash of creativity, I have subtracted, added, embellished, substituted — and gained.

For a rational, relatively mature non-crackpot, I have fallen for every screeching headline about every "diet discovery" guaranteed to remove "unwanted pounds" within a matter of days — except perhaps for the one that advocates sitting in the tub (and I admit to saving the ad for that one!). After twenty-plus years of doing the Diets Gavotte, I have been struck by a thundering truth: The "sensible," nutritious, non-fad diets are the ones that bring long-term success.

Now I have found one that works for me — a daily weigh-in program with supportive counselors who know what it is all about because they've been there, a food plan that emphasizes broiled fish and chicken, a variety of vegetables and fruits, a protein supplement, vitamins, calcium and lots of water. This, combined with the principles learned in a weight-losing group, make for a double-zappo effort.

List two disciplines which help you lose:

_____

_____

What kind of a trimdown works best for
you: _____

_____

_____

Vow here to stay with it.

I so vow. _____
(your name)

You are bendable once more at six
and better able to pick up sticks —
(or anything else you might have
dropped: your toothbrush under the
basin, a deck of cards while learning a
new shuffle, a bottle's worth of vitamin
capsules, the Sunday paper, a set of
baby blocks, your glove on an escala-
tor, clothes pins, a box of rubber bands,
your wind-scattered thesis,
daisies in a field,
your cigar box full
of fix-it supplies.)

Onward and downward! To . . .

227

7

(come eleven?)

Your boss notices.
Equivalent: A watermelon in August.

I am learning to picture myself thin — really create a sharp mental image of myself thinner. It is hard work, especially when the mirror persists in telling me that I am porky. I look down and pretend to see thin thighs instead of shirred ones; a long, unbroken wrist line without a natural bracelet; a hand, no longer dimpling at the knuckles, with a visible fan of bones; sharper knees; sharper ankles; and shinbones that are becoming ridges instead of indents. There really is beginning to be a difference. I see it first in the wrist — which I stare at appreciatively quite often.

I can picture myself doing things I have always wanted to do. Hiking along a mountain trail where the air is thin and clear, wearing a backpack. Riding a horse (a fat old waterbed of a horse will do just fine). Climbing a very small Alp or a not-so-Grand Teton. Now with a thinner body that carries out my biddings without groaning, I can at least regard such activity as a remote possibility and not simply a joke.

I have added ten more to my morning sit-ups.

List a few activities that you look forward to doing — once you are thinner _____

_____

_____

_____

_____

I can do more with less.

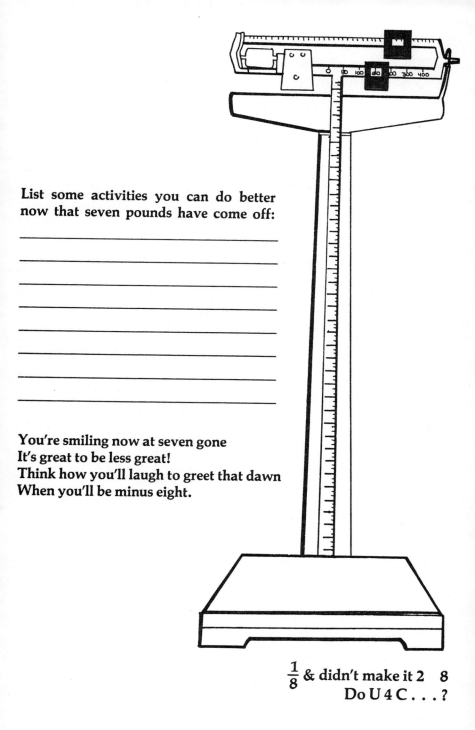

List some activities you can do better now that seven pounds have come off:

_____

_____

_____

_____

_____

_____

_____

You're smiling now at seven gone
It's great to be less great!
Think how you'll laugh to greet that dawn
When you'll be minus eight.

$\frac{1}{8}$ & didn't make it 2   8
Do U 4 C . . . ?

**You fit into a size smaller T-shirt.
(Buy yourself one, on sale, as a reward.)**
Equivalent: A man's bowling ball.

Made it through the weekend without gaining, and even managed to lose a little. Maybe I have at long last stopped thinking of eating on Sunday as the brightness at the end of a six-day tunnel, my well-deserved prize at the end of a tough week. Vague stirrings of that ancient "food is a reward" idea still persist unless I concentrate fully on making Sunday like any other day.

Have I finally learned, too, not to bow down to the dietary tyranny of a taskmaster Saturday? The whirl of Saturday's stevedore household-upkeep jobs, along with its scruffy parade of young ruffians banging in and out of doors and demanding sweets, has been known to throw me into a nervous binge. Hard labor is habitually rewarded with extra amounts of food, isn't it? Not necessarily. Now I look upon an active Saturday's work load as a boon, a chance to burn a few extra calories.

Of course, weekends are not much like ordinary middle-of-the-week days. But if I am going to get anywhere on this major thindown of mine, I will have to hold to the same weekday disciplines that are bringing success: Keeping my weight-losing plan at the top of my priority list. Spending minimal time fussing over food preparation in the kitchen. Daily readings to keep my thoughts in the right place. Daily exercise. Daily requests for spiritual fortitude. A prayer and a plan.

And — oh, yes — I'll buy a bag of apples for those ruffians, those slurpers of sweets, lest they inspire me also to so slurp.

**A weekend does not have to mean
the end of the weak!**

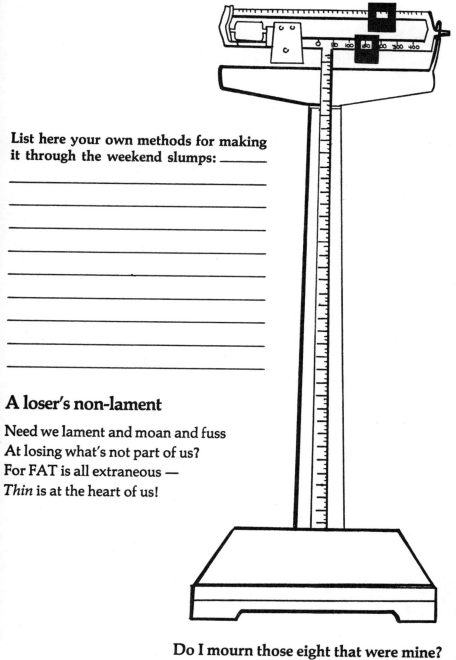

List here your own methods for making it through the weekend slumps: _____

_____
_____
_____
_____
_____
_____
_____
_____

A loser's non-lament

Need we lament and moan and fuss
At losing what's not part of us?
For FAT is all extraneous —
Thin is at the heart of us!

Do I mourn those eight that were mine?
Never! Now let's work toward . . .

9

Your carpool notices — and cheers you on.

Equivalent: The P-Z volume of the *Compact Edition of the Oxford English Dictionary* (plus four ounces extra).

I myself have not changed very much — or so it seems to me — but my clothes are growing! I am buttoning buttons that once were nearly pulled from their cloth bed from sheer strain. And the armholes — those most discouraging gauges of overweight — miraculously no longer bind. Nothing has brought me closer to tears than the binding armhole. The sleeve that could not be peeled on above the elbow or the telltale wrinkles across the upper arm.

I am careful not to set goals that stretch the limits of reality, such as: *certainly* I will fit into a whole size smaller by next weekend, and will, most surely, be able to wear that new pair of dawn-blue pants. Great if I make it. A stalling blow to my impetus if I don't. Sizing up the situation — and my body — realistically, it may take me two weeks to work my way into that pair of pants. And, even then, dawn blue may not be the most sensational color to cover my rear. Small goals are fine and encouraging. The trick is to sort out the possible from the not quite possible and set my sights accordingly.

A Day at a Time. I take some of my literary snacks daily from the book of the same name — and from Jeane Eddy Westin's *The Thin Book.* They bolster my morale and add steadiness to my commitment.

232

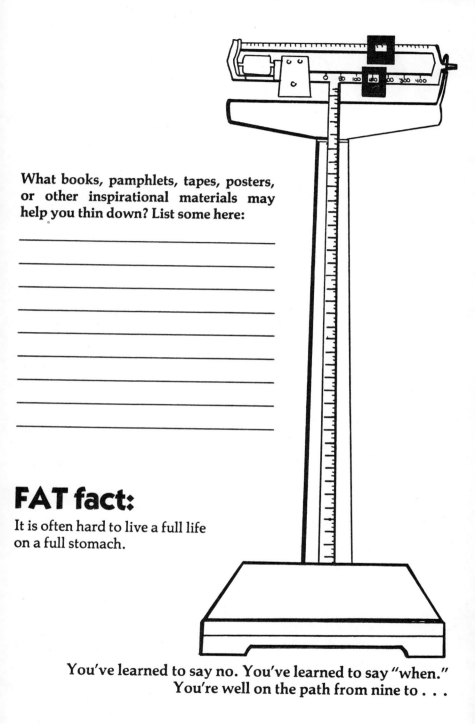

What books, pamphlets, tapes, posters, or other inspirational materials may help you thin down? List some here:

_____

_____

_____

_____

_____

_____

_____

_____

FAT fact:

It is often hard to live a full life on a full stomach.

You've learned to say no. You've learned to say "when."
You're well on the path from nine to . . .

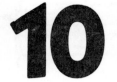

The nurse in your doctor's office notices.

Equivalent: Enough patching compound to spread an eighth-inch layer over ten square feet of wall.

Why are we so conditioned to think in tens — in ten-pound increments of loss? A seven and a half pounds loss may be every bit as important as ten. But whenever we hit a ten-pound marker, we send up balloons and shouts of thanksgiving. We bring on the trumpets and the drums, unfurl the banners and, generally, whoop for joy. Today I whooped for joy!

Why is it, too, that passing a ten-pound milestone seems to be the most slippery crossing of all? I have met my mini-goal of ten, twenty, thirty, forty or more, so it's time for celebration. E-e-e-e-asy does it. "Celebrate" is not a synonym for "eat." Moments of accomplishments, I am finding, are moments to watch out for.

My son fell for a wayside deli's concoction — a huge, hat-shaped meringue blooming out of a pastry — and brought it home with magi tenderness. Wonder of wonders, I am not even slightly tempted by it, probably because it is so enormous and steep that it looks more like a lampshade than a dessert.

I know better, however, than to taste it. Whenever I have made the mistake of putting sugar on my tongue, after weeks of refined-sugar-abstinence, it has had a rather unpleasant, sharp, too-sweet taste. I am aware though, that at the second bite, that foreign sharpness would mellow. And after the third, I would not stop until the one hundred and third! Although many seem to be able to spoon sugar into themselves with no ill effects, I, for one, can't. Besides the inevitable weight gain from eating too much of it, I detect an odd moodiness in myself and scary feeling that I may not be able to stop once I start consuming it.

It has taken me half a lifetime to rap this simple concept, based on my own experience, into my somewhat thick head — a head that is still, no doubt, the ballroom for those illusionary sugar plums.

I believe that I am a thin person.
My thinness has just not manifested
itself fully as yet.

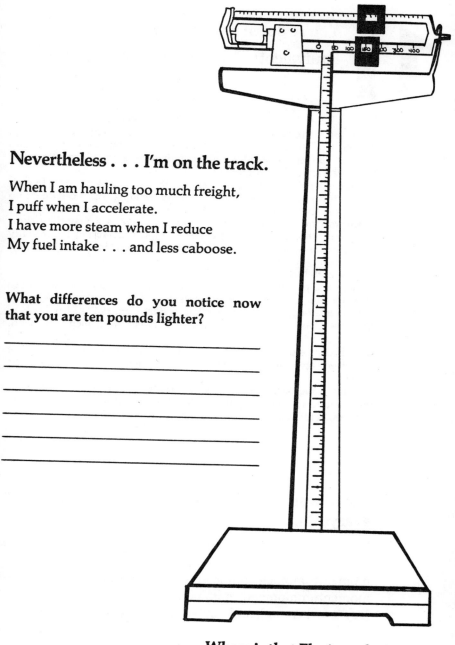

Nevertheless . . . I'm on the track.

When I am hauling too much freight,
I puff when I accelerate.
I have more steam when I reduce
My fuel intake . . . and less caboose.

What differences do you notice now that you are ten pounds lighter?

_____
_____
_____
_____
_____

Where is that Elysian, elusive . . .

235

11

You're down a whole size.
Equivalent: Thirteen copies of this book.

I can eek into a size smaller. What a joy to uncloset items of clothing from the bottoms of boxes and the dim, nether regions of storage closets — just to see what I might refit. A collection of old (and smaller) clothes are an album of remembrances every bit as bittersweet as a scrapbook of photographs.

Here is a pair of shorts I skinned into the year I was married. In fact, I wore them astride a dusty burro on my wedding trip. I can't get into those yet, but I will, I will. Here, too, is a pair of belled slacks, leftovers from the *Yellow Submarine* era. Here is a maternity dress with that awful cutout porthole. Here, limply proclaiming the frivolity of earlier days, is a costume worn when I danced in a Moulin Rouge number in a benefit follies. The state of my legs now (brawny) would make a high-kick either an impossibility or an obscenity.

Here is a pair of overalls spattered with a few spots of rooster red from the first time we painted the outside of the house.

Here is a believe-it-or not number, a skirt from 1947's New Look — volumes of brown velveteen hung on a twenty-four-inch waistband, meant to swing ankle length just above a gleam of gold sandals and dark-brown stockings. I had intended to upholster a chair in that velveteen, after my own upholstery prevented me from hooking the waist.

After losing thirty pounds, a whopping garage sale will be in order. I will start now, bagging up the clothes that are a size too big. If I get rid of them, I cut off my re-entry into a state of FAT.

If you want to lose weight, momentum is everything.

Momentum means moment to moment-to
moment-to-moment-to-moment-to-moment-to
momenttomomenttomomenttomomenttomomentto
momentummomentummomentummomentum
(say it fast enough and you've got momentum)

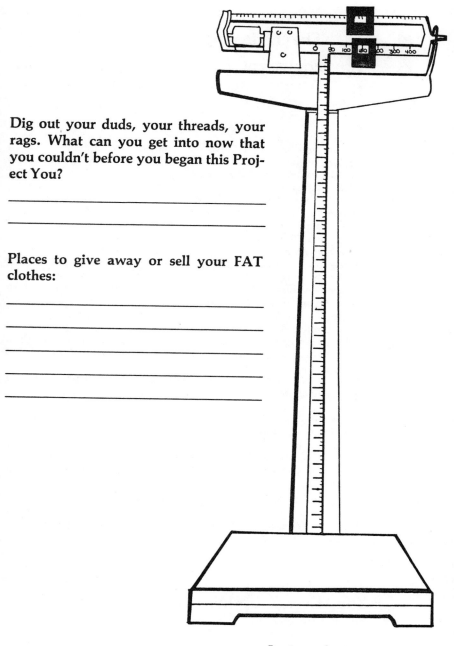

Dig out your duds, your threads, your rags. What can you get into now that you couldn't before you began this Project You?

_____

_____

Places to give away or sell your FAT clothes:

_____

_____

_____

_____

Let's make it an even . . .

12

The children notice.
Equivalent: Sixty-four hardboiled Grade A eggs, unpeeled.

I said I would be honest. So I must confess to a food slip — yes, a daughter's birthday cheek by jowl with a major holiday and a houseful of mouths to feed provided irresistible stimuli. Just when I thought I was finally in control. So I must have been staring at this page for six days when it should have required about three.

What happened to my commitment? What happened to my triumph at being able to zip into a whole size smaller — with a few bulges and pinches, but "into" nevertheless? Too much triumph? Too much smugness? Too much of feeling "aha-I'm-on-top-of-this-weight-thing?"

A few more dress rehearsals, an imaginary preview of the tempting situation in order to practice my no-thankses might have deterred the fall. **Candles blown out. No thank-you to the celebratory baked dessert. Scrape the frosted scraps into the cat's dish — be quick — or into the garbage with the smelly grapefruit rinds and coffee grounds.** Even I, the human electric pig, the infallible Disposall, probably will not be tempted at garbage. Although, at the height of my food addiction, I had been known to lift an untainted sweeting from the top of the heap and consume it. Sick?

The only blessed aspect of a slip is that if I hop right back on the diet wagon, deviation from my eating plan does not have to turn into a lost weekend or a week-long disaster. The weight added by a short-term slip **can** come off fast, especially if I do not succumb to such negative self-scolding as, "Oh, woe, I guess I'll never learn." "I must just be destined to be the captive of my compulsions forever," or "I'll probably NEVER be thin." A "poor FAT me" attitude results in lower regard for myself which makes it possible for "don't care" to take over.

I will remember that a morning slip does not have to mean a whole day devoted to FAT-making. A Friday night slip does not have to mean a catastropic weekend. Thin is worth striving for. So I am one pound down after a week instead of a more respectable two and a half pounds or so. The direction is downward. That's what matters.

You can walk upstairs without stopping to rest on the landing.

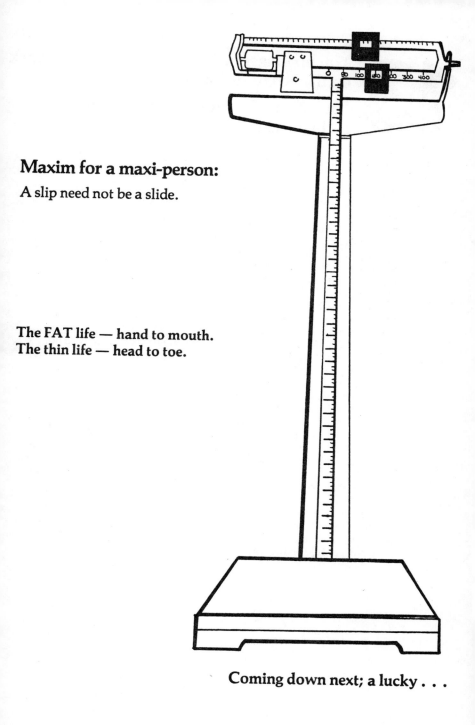

Maxim for a maxi-person:
A slip need not be a slide.

The FAT life — hand to mouth.
The thin life — head to toe.

Coming down next; a lucky . . .

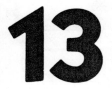

13

You no longer have to roll over on your back on the bed to pull on your socks.

Equivalent: Twenty-six LP recordings in their jackets.

What does the word "big" mean to me? What do I associate with largeness? Stretch the memory back. At the very first, "big" meant grown up, powerful, in control. It described a glorious, mature, all-ruling adult state. "Big" persons were the law-givers, the mediators, the soothers, the keepers of knowledge. They did giant deeds on athletic fields. They stood as tall as God himself in the pulpits, or so it seemed to my childish, scaled-down vision. In doctor's offices, they loomed huge and white-coated, dispensers both of pain and good humor.

"Big" also meant kind and gentle and ultimately wise, like my father, who stood six feet four and a half inches tall in his stocking feet. My unquestioned goal was to be a "big person." All things would be possible "when I got big," which I proceeded systematically to do.

Did I start back in those days eating my way to bigness? Where, along the way, did "big" turn into FAT?

Big is beautiful when it applies to mountains, hearts, spaces, sky, bank accounts, the moon, trees, bosoms, blossoms, melons, lawns, the sound of symphony orchestras, strawberries, yachts and pumpkins.

Big is not beautiful when it comes to automobiles, grizzly bears who hang around campgrounds, superhighways, jumbo jets, enrollment in college classes, crowds, backpacks, warts, a river spilling over its banks, forest fires, baskets full of laundry, hordes of insects — and the extra, useless collections of pounds which many of us designed-to-be-thin humans carry around with us.

If I give in to the "big is beautiful" school, I am a defeatist. Whatever I — and my little spoon — have made big, I can also make small. I do not hold with the obvious discrimination against OWs. I do believe in self-acceptance and a positive self-image. But I also believe in **trying.** "Big is beautiful" on the way to being smaller.

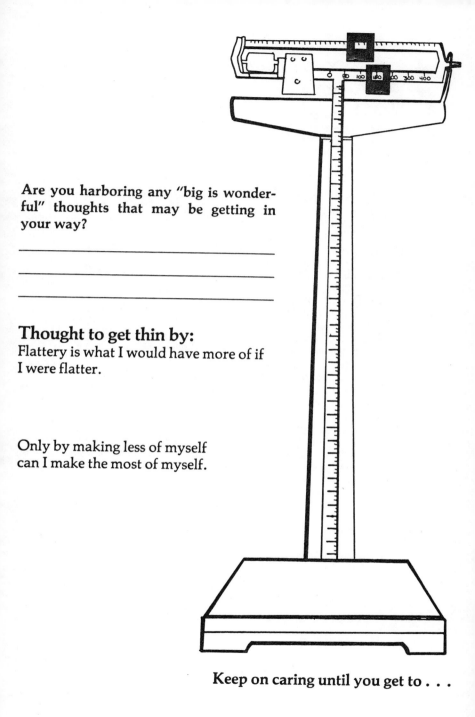

Are you harboring any "big is wonderful" thoughts that may be getting in your way?

_____

_____

_____

Thought to get thin by:

Flattery is what I would have more of if I were flatter.

Only by making less of myself can I make the most of myself.

Keep on caring until you get to . . .

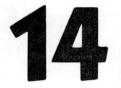

14

You can feel your collar bones.

Equivalent: One stone (think of a big one), a measure of weight in Great Britain.

Why am I so fascinated with what spare people eat? It borders on an obsession, an over-concern which I had hoped would disappear as I became less and less interested in what *anybody* ate, including myself. Why do I peer over the tops of restaurant booths to check out what that human stork seated at the bench in back of me is shoving nonchalantly into her face? I admit some residual resentment at the abandon with which she is putting away a multi-colored, buttressed and balconied frozen dessert after a plateful of fried things. Even though I am on the way to becoming normal myself, this wonder persists. How can a few of the ultra-thin keep on this way, consuming calories by the hundreds? I take some comfort in the fact that several skinny overconsumers do, given enough time and unchanging habits of indulgence, begin to blow up like the rest of us, to their astonishment.

These ex-storks make up a special sub-group of overweights; they fall into the surprised-by-FAT category. I, on the other hand, have given myself plenty of time to get used to my FAT. The slow build-up did away with any element of surprise!

Now I am heading for the surprised-by-thin category instead.

I will try not to compare myself to the thin ones who can overeat blithely, without gaining. I will, instead, find my inspiration among those who so happily startle me with their successful weight losses. Let *them* be my models.

Comparing selves with those who are slimmer
Can light our sparks or make them dimmer.
Abandon any sad proclivities
To be undermined by relativities!

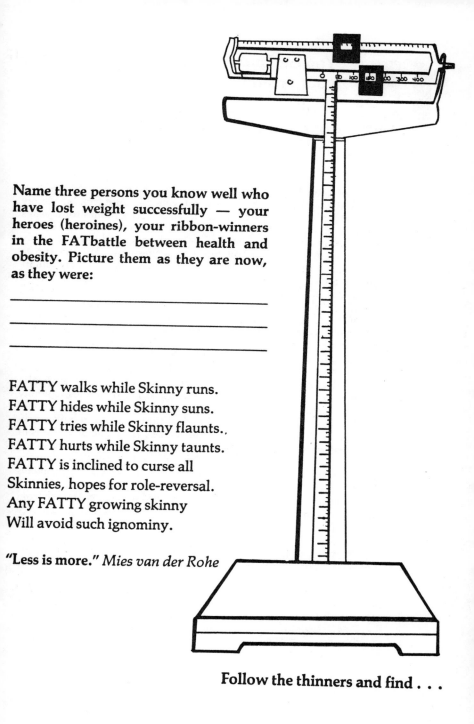

Name three persons you know well who have lost weight successfully — your heroes (heroines), your ribbon-winners in the FATbattle between health and obesity. Picture them as they are now, as they were:

_____

_____

_____

FATTY walks while Skinny runs.
FATTY hides while Skinny suns.
FATTY tries while Skinny flaunts..
FATTY hurts while Skinny taunts.
FATTY is inclined to curse all
Skinnies, hopes for role-reversal.
Any FATTY growing skinny
Will avoid such ignominy.

"Less is more." *Mies van der Rohe*

Follow the thinners and find . . .

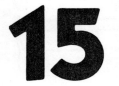

15

You can buckle a sandal without cutting off your breathing.

Equivalent: A pumpkin
for an enormous Jack o'Lantern.

Now that I am thinner, I am struck by just how much my FATness pinched the family budget. (This is no reveling-in-guilt trip, but simply a look at a now-changing reality.) Eleven dollars a month for a year's membership in a spa that I was too humiliated to use because I looked like a shortly-after-high-noon shadow — all squat and black — in my leotard. I-hate-to-tell-you-how-much to a masseuse called in for an occasional (very occasional) drubbing. An extra thirty to forty dollars a month added to grocery and meat bills, just to feed my food habit. Frozen diet dinners that sat in the freezer and frosted up while I carefully avoided them. Tankfuls of diet pop. The cost of outsize clothing. And so many shoes, to replace the rowboat-shaped footgear that I stretched out at the top or wore down at the sole in a month's time — with all that gravity at work. An added thirty dollars a month on a life insurance policy because of my "special" classification.

Then there were: psychologists, weight counselors, nutrition experts, doctors, diet clubs, diet recipe books, diet magazines, health club memberships, home "gyms," exercise belts, treadmills, shimmy machines, jump ropes, pedal-in-place bicycles, rubber suits, rubber waistbands, rubber girdles, diet "candy," fill-you-up-with-bulk crackers, lecithin, liquid protein, diet "milk shakes," a couple of versions of a diet meal-in-a-can, a couple of kinds of meal-in-a-bar, running shoes, sweat (I mean literally) suits, hypnotists' tapes, hypnotists' seminars, a gadget that counts your bites, make-up (to make up for problems elsewhere).

And the accessories: Filmy scarves intended to distract the eye from the over-all immensity of my image. A few compellingly chunky baubles ditto. A huge chiffon peony that made me look like a potted Mother's Day plant or a cow dining on a meadow blossom. Sweaters, shawls, capes, drapes — any extra layer to hide my *own* extra layers.

Moneys thus spent could have paid the best part of a college freshman's tuition!

Anything that worked was worth every grudgingly given cent! But nothing *really* worked until I began to take responsibility for my own HEW (health, education and welfare), until I began to count less on gimmicks and more on God, until I stopped searching for the Aha-so-*that's*-it! "reason" behind my overweight and treated the symptom — FAT. The "why's" were bigger than my stomach (which was big)!

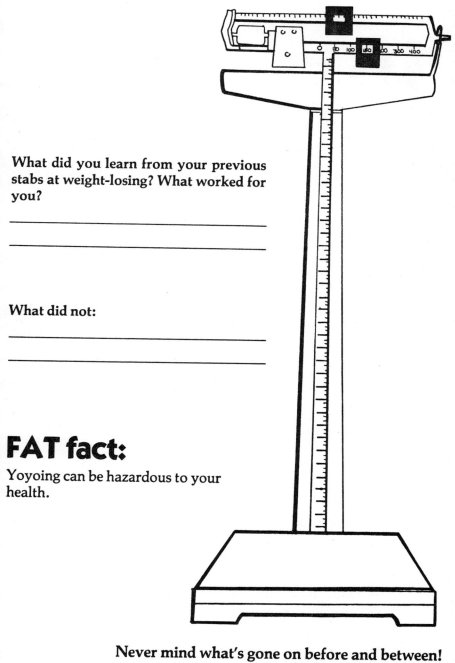

What did you learn from your previous stabs at weight-losing? What worked for you?

_____

_____

What did not:

_____

_____

FAT fact:

Yoyoing can be hazardous to your health.

**Never mind what's gone on before and between!
You've lost a laudable . . .**

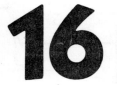

16 You have a waist again. Borrow a hole-puncher. Your belts need new buckle holes.

Equivalent: Four packages of lawn fertilizer — enough to cover 4,000 square feet (or 2,400 square feet in California).

I feel fragile, breakable — which is somewhat laughable, because I am actually far from it. In fact, sturdy would be an apt descriptive term. I am enjoying a feeling of "running on empty." It makes me know I am getting somewhere.

Maybe this lightness is synonymous with joy! Like an Aubusson tapestry, like a modern soft sculpture, I have two bathing suits taped to my closet door. One is the full-skirted, full-breasted, full-bodied model bought during my Blubber-era and worn once, in the back yard when nobody was around. One is a meager rainbow of a bikini which I plan to wear some day. It's a dieter's game: Just how little will I be able to put on and still be covered? This is not to say that I would ever venture beyond the four walls of my bedroom clad only in a couple of bandanas. Probably not, since already I am adorned with such personal accessories as stretch marks and thighs that drape like Roman curtains now that I am depleting them of their FAT. Tightening exercises are in order! I am overripe for such scantiness. The bikini is merely a gauge — along with my scale, my mirror, before-and-after photographs, the bones I am beginning to feel through my padding, the remarks of friends, the reactions of fellow dieters.

A private rhyme

Bikini on the closet door —
It hangs there as my "carrot,"
But only my scale and I will know
If I ever choose to wear it.

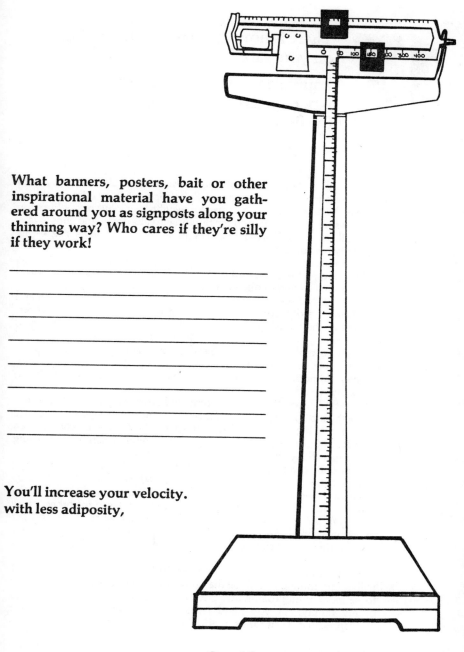

What banners, posters, bait or other inspirational material have you gathered around you as signposts along your thinning way? Who cares if they're silly if they work!

_____

_____

_____

_____

_____

_____

_____

You'll increase your velocity.
with less adiposity,

Good for you! You've shed sixteen.
going on . . .

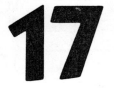

There is now room for your lap dog on your lap.
Equivalent: Five hundred and fifty-four No. 6 brass casting sinkers for fishermen.

If this treatise seems single-minded to the point of absurdity, it has to be. The moment any concerns — global or cosmic or even neighborhood — begin to boot the business of weight-losing out of my life's top priority spot, my motivation for thinning breaks down and ebbs away. After all, how can I presume to complain over the body's size — the unseemly heft of just one insignificant human — when the Middle East is in an uproar, man-launched objects are slithering from their orbits and crashing among us, and other people in other parts of the world are stick-limbed and swollen-bellied from starvation?

In the light of such matters, the state of my body and my health and well-being hardly seem worth such concentrated effort. However, looking at the world's problems — and my own — from a practical, less sweeping point of view, I conclude that whatever contribution I am able to make will be greater if I am smaller. I will have more energy, more optimism, more regard for myself. I will be less snared in my own do-nothing fantasies and less haunted by worries of incapacitating overweight.

As a FAT, I spend too much time and strength just thinking about where the next pound might come from — and how to get rid of it once it comes. A big "what if": What if all the FATs of this country (an estimated 60 per cent of the adult populace) who presently are wasting hours upon hours in self-pity and self-recrimination over their bigger-than-normal condition used those same hours in various causes for human betterment? If even half of that 60 percent, or 93,102,000 Americans, worry about their weight for — say — a total of a half-hour per day, that could mean 46,551,000 hours freed for other, more important things. The only way to free up that worry time and get something done is for us FATs to get thin and stop frittering away our time fretting over weight problems. Human betterment begins with my own.

If I'm feeling a tad guilty about the selfishness of my diet program, I will do my thinmost to erase that guilt. I must be selfish today in order to be more giving tomorrow. Stick by me, all you underfed members of my family, all you good friends whose supper invitations are unreciprocated. Wait for us, world. We'll do more for you thinner.

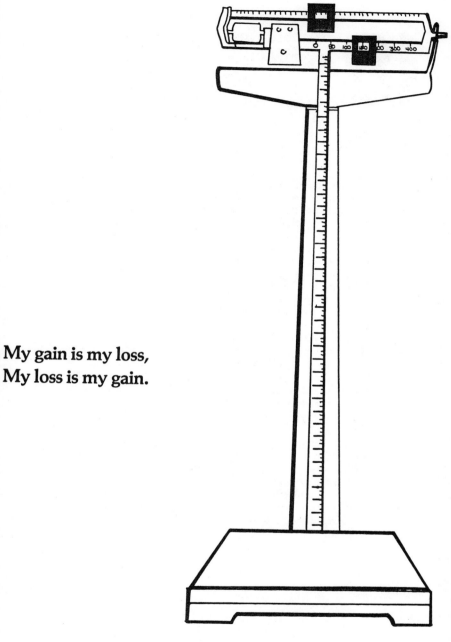

My gain is my loss,
My loss is my gain.

Be a good loser and move on to . . .

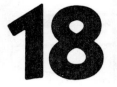

Your life insurance agent smiles upon you.

Equivalent: The first six volumes (A to Civil Law) of the Encyclopedia Americana, 1965 edition.

Soft or tough? When I was an extremely FAT FAT (I am now a moderately FAT FAT). I took some small comfort in categorizing FATfolk into arbitrary subgroups: Soft FATS and tough FATS. Soft FATS I envisioned as loungers and do-littles, pillowy types who reclined on chaises lounges and popped bonbons. I linked soft FATS with leisure and lack of muscle tone. A soft FAT frequented fancy restaurants. I pictured the white linen napkin tucked firmly under a multiplicity of chins. I have never known such a creature, but conjuring up this fluffy-FAT stereotype somehow made me feel better, *I* was definitely not one of *those.*

I was a tough FAT. Tough FATS were solid, with plenty of muscle to brace the excess pounds and cart them around. A tough FAT, in spite of the handicap of overweight, does not give up easily, but keeps right on swinging through life headlong, stalwartly meeting challenges with a relatively calm exterior — while eating too much.

Somehow a tough FAT condition was, to me, less reprehensible and more excusable than a soft FAT condition. I automatically classified other overweights as mostly fluff or mostly tough. Although it was not okay to be FAT, it was more okay to be a tough FAT than a fluffy, soft FAT.

Such categorizing was all part of my web of excuses. The truth is: FAT is FAT, and that is that. Not a sin. Not a wrong. Not a moral or ethical issue, As a fact, I can deal with it. If FATness gets mixed up with a shaky psyche, a feeble character, weakness of will or any other human complexities, it comes much harder to cope with. Some of us simply consume more food than we need to keep us running efficiently. Some of us need to change a few patterns. Plain and simple. A day at a time.

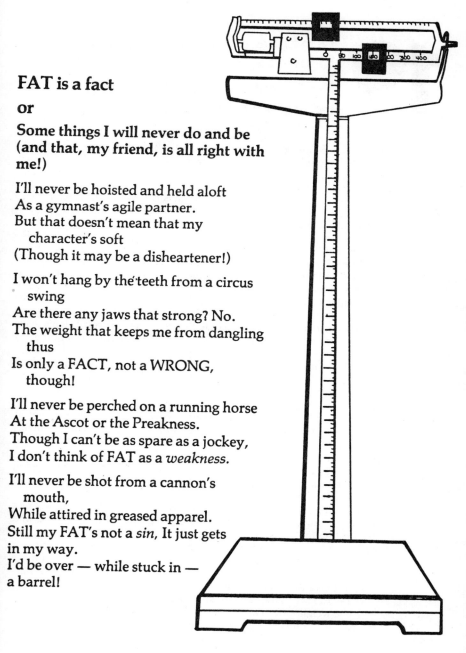

FAT is a fact

or

Some things I will never do and be (and that, my friend, is all right with me!)

I'll never be hoisted and held aloft
As a gymnast's agile partner.
But that doesn't mean that my
   character's soft
(Though it may be a disheartener!)

I won't hang by the teeth from a circus
   swing
Are there any jaws that strong? No.
The weight that keeps me from dangling
   thus
Is only a FACT, not a WRONG,
   though!

I'll never be perched on a running horse
At the Ascot or the Preakness.
Though I can't be as spare as a jockey,
I don't think of FAT as a *weakness*.

I'll never be shot from a cannon's
   mouth,
While attired in greased apparel.
Still my FAT's not a *sin*, It just gets
in my way.
I'd be over — while stuck in —
a barrel!

**Coming up next:
a fantastically fine . . .**

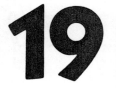

Don't look now, but you're being followed by a FAT shadow.

Equivalent: a turkey big enough to feed the whole family plus an aunt and two cousins.

I am being followed by a FAT shadow. I fully expect to look down and see a bulging inky blob trailing after me in the sunlight. Why, now that I am thinner, do I still feel FAT? Have I forgotten how to feel thin? Did I ever know?

I may have to learn the actual physical feeling of FATness or thinness, quite apart from the statement which runs and reruns in my head, "Oh, Lord, I'm so FAT!"

I may even still see a FAT self in the mirror, though all the data proves that I have at last become thinner.

My FAT shadow sometimes keeps me from making the most of my thin self. I still expect the barrel reflection in the store window, the turned-off glances of passersby. I still head for the navy blues and the right sides of the racks where the "larger" sizes droop. I have never really lost my fears of loneliness, and, yes, believe it or not, of starvation. I still hide from people in the grocery stores. I don't want them to see what I put in the cart. Now, if other shoppers bother to look, they will find mostly greenery and fresh fruits and vegetables there. Nothing at all to be sneaky about. Quite a change from the days when I piled it with blank white bags and boxes from the bakery department! But FAT habits cling. They can be as hard to lose as the weight itself.

The time to start retraining myself to become a thin person is not at the end of a successful trimdown, but during it. I can begin to practice *living* thin at that wondrous moment when I make the commitment to *become* thin.

I need to practice looking at people eye-to-eye instead of dropping my gaze to my feet. (Yes, they *are* becoming less like loaves of bread popping over the pan tops.)

Since thin means active, I need to add activity to my life — an extra half-a-parking-lot's stride between the place where I leave the car and my destination, a walk for walking's sake (not purely to get some-where), a new sport, a new dance, a new exercise. I can add activities as I feel ready to take them on. If I don't yet feel prepared to don the swimwear and plunge into a routine of daily laps in a pool, I can start with a covered-up walk or jog.

I need to make sure I am not still walking FAT. Some ex-FATs, even with the weight off, waddle. This calls for learning to walk thin. I will try for less roll and pitch, more evenness in my stride — a taller, straighter, floating feeling.

I will act with thin independence, thin self-confidence, thin control, thin discipline. If I was a scatterbrained FAT, I will be an organized thin. I will act thin, even before I get there. After all, I am on the way.

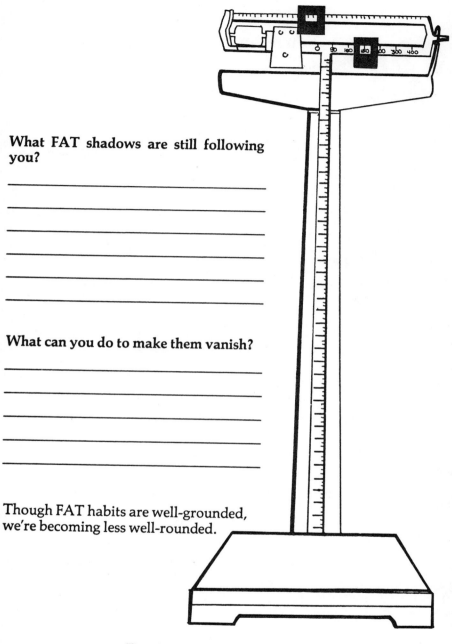

What FAT shadows are still following you?

_____

_____

_____

_____

_____

_____

What can you do to make them vanish?

_____

_____

_____

_____

_____

Though FAT habits are well-grounded, we're becoming less well-rounded.

Don't stop now: You've almost made it to . . .

253

20

You're down another entire size.
Equivalent: A five-week-old hog.

Whew. Passed the almost-twenty-pound plateau, where I had cooled my heels and tapped my fingers impatiently for more than a week, wondering if I was destined to stall forever with one third of the way still to go. A little extra burst of activity helped to flip me off that plateau and send me downward again. I added five more to my daily sit-ups, coaxed my good mate into an hour and half of after-work singles on a tennis court and started to jog (only about a quarter of a mile to start with). Just a slow run a couple of times around the nearby street loop, an activity usually undertaken early in the morning before my unavoidable bouncing catches the eyes of any curious nonrunners.

A discovery — or rather, a theory suspected and self-tested: If I exercise more, I do not seem to be as hungry. This is not science talking — simply the instinct of just one FAT who is wont to snatch at any constructive flicker of possible truth that can help. All I know is — I'm unstuck and on my way again. Praise be.

Crazy thought for the day for thinning parents: Treat your supplier — your hand — as a toddler, an into-everything two-year-old, requiring constant vigilance and frequent, emphatic, timely NO's.

There is only one road to FAT — through the mouth. If I were a military strategist, I would find the obvious solution: Cut off the supply route. And win the FAT battle.

I have control over my elbow.
I have control over my hand.
I have control over my mouth.
That is all the control I need.

How simple the laws of cause and effect.
From table to mouth — the route is direct.

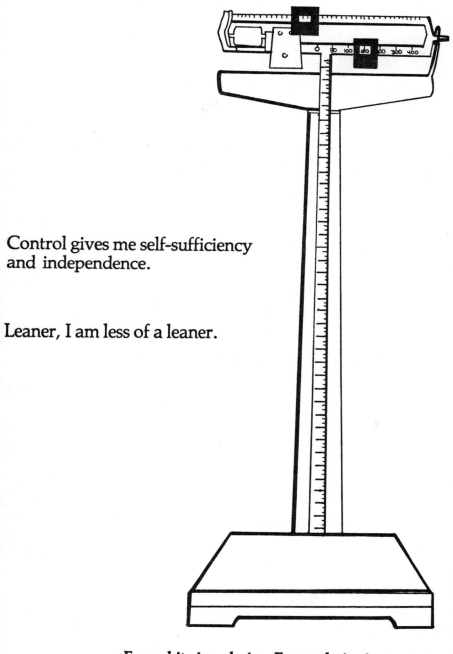

Control gives me self-sufficiency
and independence.

Leaner, I am less of a leaner.

**Every bite is a choice. Every choice is my own.
Choose to move on to . . .**

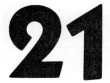

21

An old friend stops you on the street and tells you how great you look.

Equivalent: triplets.

A small error in judgment — mine — makes me feel not very good about myself.

With negative thoughts gathering like stormclouds in the southwest, I know I have to do something — quick — to keep them from blowing away my diet program. A few affirming words are in order:

> *I am a thin person.*
> I am not hungry.
> Three regular meals a day are plenty for me — I don't need to eat between meals.
> *I am a thin person.*
> I am much more interested in (fill in your own activity here — reading, swimming, dancing, woodworking, painting, whatever) than I am in eating.
> I like lettuce and green beans.
> I like broiled fish.
> I like to run.
> *I am a thin person.*
> *Yes, indeed, I am, after all, a thin person.*

I find it absolutely amazing that I really am beginning to believe these positive statements. Are they tricks? Am I snowing myself? I think not, because all of these words have a root of truth. They are all possible. If they are possible, they may be likely. If they are likely, they may be probable. If they are probable, they may actually happen. And if they may happen, they will happen — if I believe positively that they will. *I am a thin person.* Saying is being.

If I *act as if* I am thin, I am beginning, right now, to live a thin life.

I am learning that a successful weight-losing plan is never *just* a plan of what to — or not to — eat. It has to involve everything that I do and that I am — what I say to myself, what I believe in, how I move, how I ease stress, how I feel, how I express how I feel, how I keep my positive purpose, and, yes, how I laugh. I am not treating only the part of me that processes food and turns it into FAT. I am treating *all* of me.

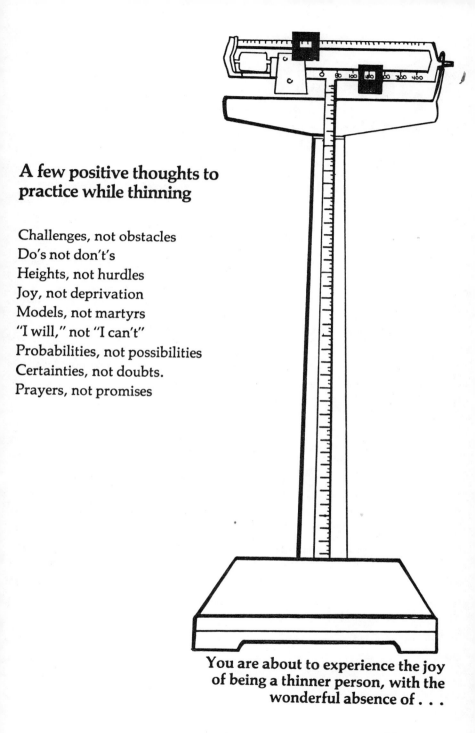

A few positive thoughts to practice while thinning

Challenges, not obstacles
Do's not don't's
Heights, not hurdles
Joy, not deprivation
Models, not martyrs
"I will," not "I can't"
Probabilities, not possibilities
Certainties, not doubts.
Prayers, not promises

You are about to experience the joy
of being a thinner person, with the
wonderful absence of . . .

22

You have doubled your walking (running) distance.
Equivalent: Half of a twin-bed mattress.

Somebody brought a paper bag to work today. Who gets turned on by a paper bag? I do. As a compulsive overeater, I can catch a glimpse of a plain white paper bag, plump and puckered shut, and think, "Bakery."

Just the sight of that bag is all it takes to roll my well-built-in inner movies of pastries-and-goo and set me to WANTING.

Not only am I trying very hard to turn off that projector which sends dreampuffs across my consciousness, but I have developed some firm, unhesitating and automatic retorts to the excuses that pop up just when I don't need them. These rationalizing phrases have been such a part of me that I need some hearty arguments against them. It is a case of instinct vs. reason. Don't care vs. care. Satisfaction of the moment vs. long-term goals.

When I hear that small coaxing voice within, I have my retorts ready to combat compulsion with control.

Go on. Look inside that bag. See if there is anything inside worth getting FAT on.

Retort: There is nothing anywhere worth getting FAT on.

Just one bite won't matter. I can sneak it in, and the scale will never notice it.

(I have, after heeding this voice, gone through a half-dozen pastry rings with holes, one bite at a time, rationalizing all the way that calories nibbled don't add up to as much as calories bolted. WRONG.)

Retort: A bite can turn into a binge.

Oh, what the heck. Nobody cares.

Retort: *I* care.

They will never know (a Sneakeater's theme song).

It doesn't matter if "they" know. *I* know. And I will like myself better if I don't listen to that wheedling voice.

Being "powerless over food" does not mean that every time I hear certain cues or see a slope-sided whipperoo with a maraschino planted like a flag on Everest, that I am going after it. It does mean that I must never let down the guard, that I can never be positive of my reaction to the temptation of food or to the words that lead me to it.

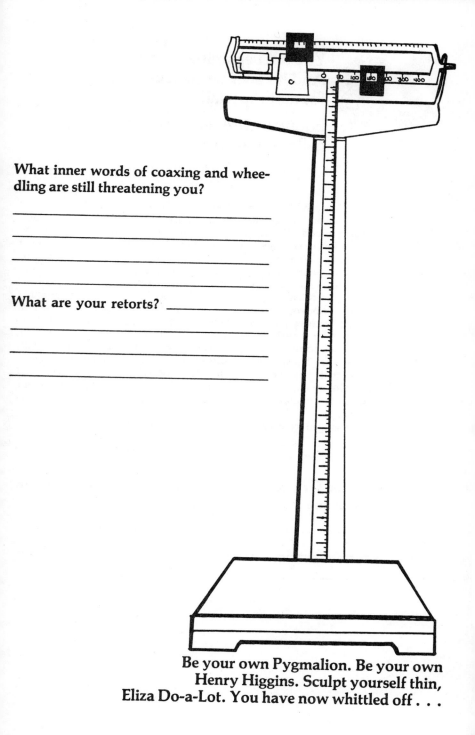

What inner words of coaxing and wheedling are still threatening you?

_____
_____
_____
_____

What are your retorts? _____

_____
_____
_____

Be your own Pygmalion. Be your own
Henry Higgins. Sculpt yourself thin,
Eliza Do-a-Lot. You have now whittled off . . .

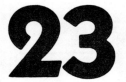

23

You are beginning to taste freedom! And it's sweeter than any soda fountain special!

Equivalent: A sump pump or, three gallons of turpentine.

Such a sense of liberation! The blessed release from obesity is like breaking out of prison, like finding a firm shore after wading in foot-grabbing muck, like flying after years of plodding uphill. Energy. Exhilaration. Happiness. I remember that old childhood trick of standing in a doorway and pressing the backs of my hands against the sides of the door frame, then stepping out and feeling my arms rise up, unbidden, like wings. I feel that same crazy lightness.

I have been transformed from a FAT setting hen into a hummingbird. God knows, I do not bear even a minimal resemblance to that whirring feathery mite. For anyone else to see the hummingbird in me will require a superior imagination, since it is quite obvious that I am still bonded to this earth by a greater-than-average gravitational pull. It's just that I *feel* hummingbird-like — a poetic, musical, magical feeling that has me identifying happily with all those trite and wonderful images of lightweight things that waft and drift through our language, from dandelion heads and dragonflies to gossamer (whatever that is).

I've changed from a rock to a sunbeam. No wonder I feel fantastic.

Describe for yourself what being thinner feels like. Learn to recognize, appreciate and sense your new thinness.

_____

_____

_____

_____

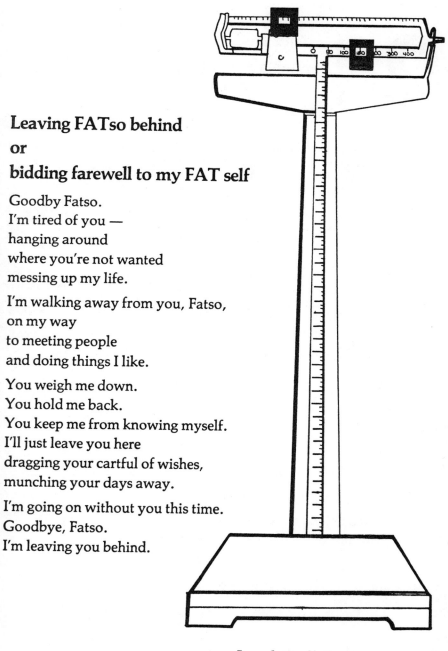

Leaving FATso behind
or
bidding farewell to my FAT self

Goodby Fatso.
I'm tired of you —
hanging around
where you're not wanted
messing up my life.

I'm walking away from you, Fatso,
on my way
to meeting people
and doing things I like.

You weigh me down.
You hold me back.
You keep me from knowing myself.
I'll just leave you here
dragging your cartful of wishes,
munching your days away.

I'm going on without you this time.
Goodbye, Fatso.
I'm leaving you behind.

Laugh it off. Lose some more.
Set your sights on . . .

24

Your ankles have stopped hurting.
Equivalent: The largest human baby
ever born (plus a few ounces).

I hoisted myself — by myself — onto a horse's back today. He was tacked up in a Western saddle, to be sure, with a convenient built-in handle. But it has been thir — well, never mind — plenty of years since I engaged in horsepersonly activities. And it was a monstrous animal, at least four stories high. (We FATS, even when trimmed down, love to exaggerate.) Once atop, I must be honest, I didn't do much except sit there and count my blessings, feeling very much as if I were on the observation tower of the IDS Building (a fifty-seven story Twin Cities skypuncher).

It's spring again. I can leave my sedentary winter ways and burrow and scrape around outside — putting in a garden, replacing the storm doors with screens, raking, blacktopping the driveway, planting a few small shrubs, hosing down the porch, tending to all those springtime weekend household needs that keep me busy and out of the kitchen. Thank heaven for spring! I actually found more thrill in a bucket of housepaint than in a bucket of deep-fried bird from the Colonel's quickie down the street. Now *that* — for me — is a healthy switch.

My own magic "open sesame"
To unlock a brand-new existence
Is just to keep working toward less of me,
With prayer and a lot of persistence.

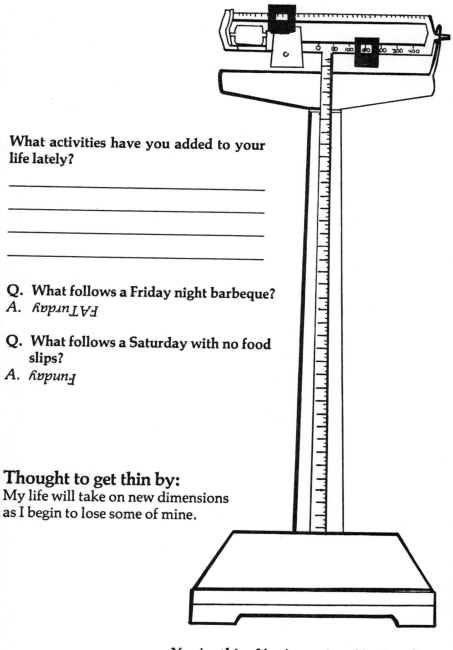

What activities have you added to your life lately?

_____

_____

_____

_____

Q. What follows a Friday night barbeque?
A. *FATurday*

Q. What follows a Saturday with no food slips?
A. *Funday*

Thought to get thin by:
My life will take on new dimensions as I begin to lose some of mine.

You're thin. You're active. You're alive,
And just over this hump is . . .

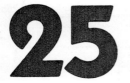

People no longer seem to look at you just because you are heavy.

Equivalent: Five hundred five-and-one-half-inch styrofoam balls.

I had the temerity to attend a school reunion, something I would never have done when I was hugely overweight. I knew that the sight of me, still padded with an abundant thirty-five pounds, would hardly bring whoops of recognition at first glance. But then, the rest of my classmates were not so immediately recognizable either, unless they had spared themselves the ravages of parenthood and stayed out of the sun.

When saying initial hellos, it was the unabashed practice to lower the gaze to the opposite bosom or lapel and read the necessary clue to that person's identity. Thank God for name tags, which wrapped up for each individual umpteen years of academic, professional and marital history. We knew in a twinkling, for example, what Mary Jones Johnson McAdam McNutt, Ph.D, M.D., had been doing to keep herself busy since graduation.

In spite of our first, superficial concern about "how we look" — about whether time had plumped us, rearranged us, dried us up, faded us, altered us in numerous small ways — it took only a few minutes for the old image of the schoolgirl with the bright hair and smooth skin to come into focus with the present, more mature picture. Until those double-images focused for me, a roomful of one-hundred-odd reuning classmates seemed to comprise a crowd of twice that many, including the leftover mental photographs of all those that once upon a collegiate time matched the names. Such a rush of images at this reunion dinner overpowered any interest I might ordinarily have in what was spread on the buffet table. In fact, I don't even remember what was served.

Imagine old food-addict me being more fascinated with the *past* (and how it has developed into the present) than the *repast!*

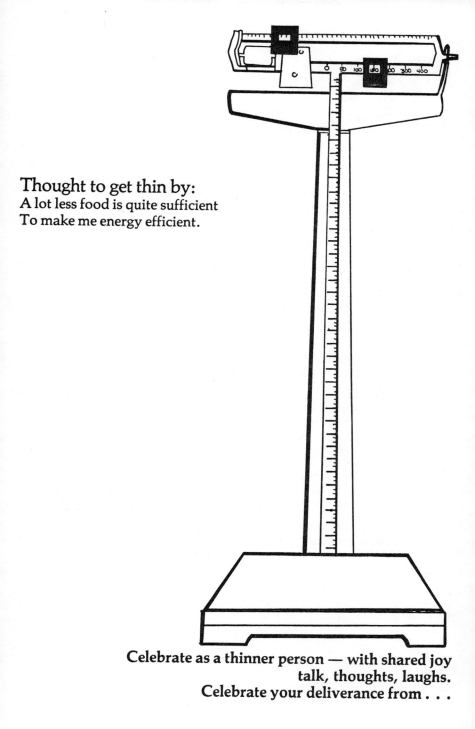

Thought to get thin by:
A lot less food is quite sufficient
To make me energy efficient.

Celebrate as a thinner person — with shared joy
talk, thoughts, laughs.
Celebrate your deliverance from . . .

265

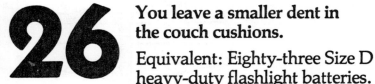

26

You leave a smaller dent in the couch cushions.

Equivalent: Eighty-three Size D heavy-duty flashlight batteries.

Seeing one-time friends who have quietly slid out of your life can mean much more than a renewal of friendships. It is a renewal of spirit. Who ever heard of a school reunion being spiritual? Such occasions are notorious for forced rowdiness that attempts to cover the shock of seeing an entire parade of smiling Dorian Grays — so suddenly (or so it seems) transformed from the tight little figures that once trotted around the campus with you or sat near you in the Rome to Roosevelt class. Spiritual because of the inner strengths that these long-ago classmates had since discovered and were happy to share. Here was an opening up of the innerness that in college days was so often guarded or costumed for a series of roles being tried for the first time.

Nostalgia clung to us like the smell of the wisteria or the tulip trees. Every familiar crack in the walks, every smoothed brass handle on a classroom building door, produced its own temporary twinge. Tramping down a pond path, a couple of us came upon a bronze, larger-than-human figure of St. Francis offering all the green of the spring forest to Heaven in a joyous sweep of his arms. A new gift to the school since our days there.

The absence of those pounds I had struggled to lose since the last time we convened was noticed and approved. And the approval set a new stamp on my commitment: I am ready again to take on a new, inspired phase in my whittling.

I appreciate my lightness — well, lighterness — on the campus dips and slopes. The calves of the legs tug, but the huffing is gone.

This thinner self merges more easily with a younger self recalled here with such sharpness. I have a new awareness of where I fit in the long scheme of things. And I am reminded with a clarity as stunning as those tea-plate-size dogwood blossoms outside the dormitory window that I fit best as a thinner, quicker-moving, busier person, less encumbered and less haunted by the burden of overweight.

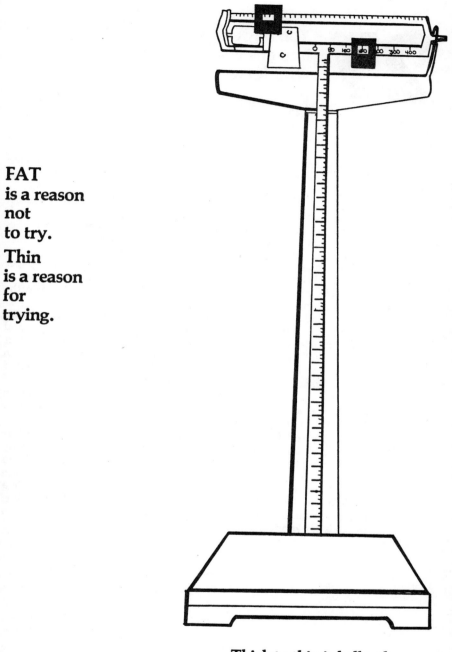

FAT
is a reason
not
to try.
Thin
is a reason
for
trying.

Thick to thin is hell to heaven.
Enjoy yourself at . . .

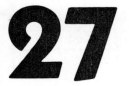

27

You buy a new bathing suit (or get into one you haven't been able to wear for a while).

Equivalent: Quadruplets.

A long holiday weekend at the lake. Vacations are fine checkpoints to discover how you are faring with your losses. How big was I last year on this holiday? What size was I wearing then?

That bikini, still an impossibility, is taped on the back of my closet door at home, waving me on to smaller things. But I do have an immediate reward for my losses to date: A new bathing suit, two sizes smaller than last year's, along with a terry cloth stretch suit to go over it. There is still plenty of flesh to cloak, but in sports clothes now I look less like an amateur handicraft project covered in Contact paper than I did last year at this time. The body is, for the first time in years, beachable, although I would still hesitate to promenade it down the street in swim wear.

Best of all, I see pride in the eyes of my good-friend-and-husband, who has seen me, quite literally, through thick and thin, for worse and for better. He is openly delighted by the changes he sees. ("Gosh, what a difference!") His eyes are the greatest mirror of all. Now I can keep up with his vacation stride. On a bicycle I can now pedal to the top of inclines (gentle ones) without turning violet and evoking mutters of concern from him. After several years of watching him cycling on ahead, or stopped and waiting for me to catch up, I can now keep up with him — a joy in itself.

Harking back to an earlier vacation, I so clearly recall looks of fear on the faces of other tourists who watched, shuddering as I hoisted my bulk to the top of a Mexican ruin and then was very nearly unable to maneuver it back down again. Has anyone ever perished from exertion on the summit of an ancient pyramid? My head swam with visions of a modern-day, hefty American woman in her grass-green culotte rolling and bouncing like a barrel down those ages-old steps — a sacrifice to the gods of overindulgence.

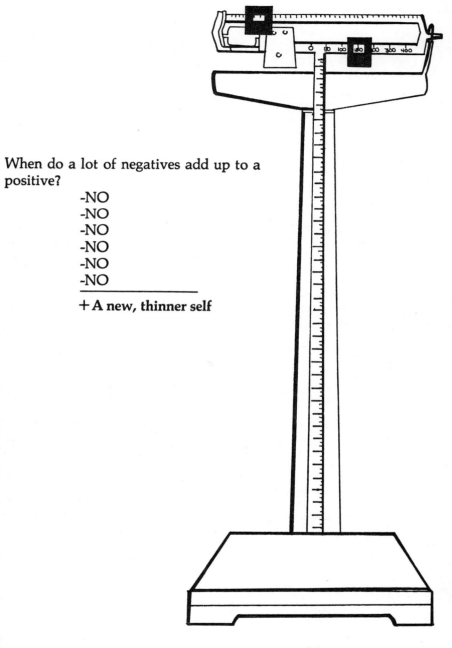

When do a lot of negatives add up to a
positive?

          -NO
          -NO
          -NO
          -NO
          -NO
          -NO
          _____
          + A new, thinner self

Yes, yes, yes to . . .

269

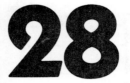 **The checkout girl at the grocery notices.**

Equivalent: A 1906 L.C. Smith & Bros. No. 2 typewriter.

There is yet another combo to unhook — eating-*and*-vacations. For me, a holiday is *not* a holiday from dieting. An adventure is not necessarily an adventure in good eating, as Duncan Hines used to say. The temptation while vacationing, is to succumb to the food specialty — whatever it is — of the place — wherever it is. And after a long history of subscribing to a when-in-Rome-eat-as-the-Romans-do theory, and giving in to every regional foodism from Key Lime Pie to Vermont maple sugar, I am convinced that there are seldom any lo-cal local food specialties. They are all FAT tourist traps (or traps for FAT tourists).

No longer do these regional foods sing their torchy songs to me. No longer do I rationalize my way into devouring them with "I may never pass this way again; it would be a shame to pass up this culinary opportunity." Once upon a FAT time, when I allowed these specialties to tempt me into consuming them, I almost always concluded that the food, once eaten, was worth neither the extra calories nor the guilt. No, thank you.

On a vacation, my husband/companion pretends to eat the way I do, kindly passing up baked offerings and other desserts in my presence, sneaking off occasionally to a soda fountain or drive-in ice cream dispensary by himself. He has no weight problem at all, although he sometimes professes to one — a sympathetic obesity. But, bless him, he is as quietly, un-naggingly dedicated to my losing goals as I am myself.

Younger members of the family have been testing out holiday restaurants, reacting with savoring 'mmmmmm's" and "wow's" to mounds, slabs, bricks, towers and temples of baked, whipped and otherwise concocted desserts. And to my surprise, perhaps for the first time in my life, I am not even tempted. I know enough, however, not to taste any of them — not even a fingerlick's worth! Give me a taste and I'll eat the whole sugary mess!

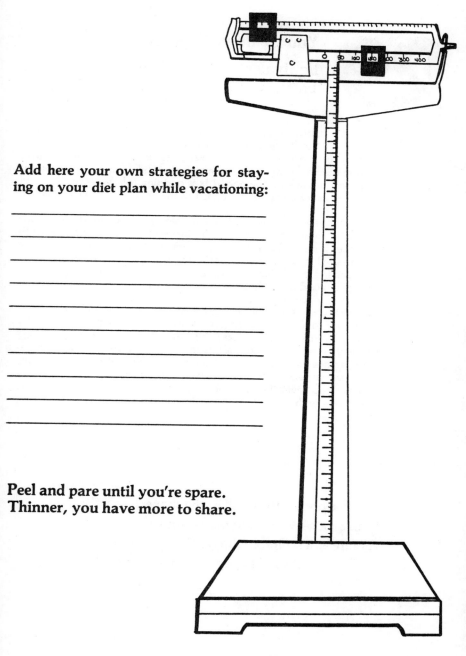

Add here your own strategies for staying on your diet plan while vacationing:

_____
_____
_____
_____
_____
_____
_____
_____
_____
_____

Peel and pare until you're spare.
Thinner, you have more to share.

You're on the brink of . . .

29

You are down three sizes in stretch knits. Equivalent: A Sears Die-Hard car battery.

I tucked a lightweight step-on scale — a friend I dare not be parted from — in the bottom of my suitcase and brought it along. The accuracy of the reading is not nearly as important as the relative position of the indicator. If I think of that scale dial as a compass, is my course holding at due north? Is it creeping (oh, woe) to the north northeast? Is it falling (all ri-i-i-ght!) to the north northwest? I need to know.

A beach scene: A scene I would have been removed from last summer at this time, by either a city block or a floor-length terrycloth tent-robe. But here I am, enjoying warm sand and the anonymity of a normal-sized body. I am not collecting stares of curiosity (and pity) from passing beach bums and bunnies while trying to maintain my feelings of good-personhood — a struggle which used to propel me to the nearest concession stand.

I watched my son's college-age friend, in a burst of post-exam-week energy, try to outrun a rabbit, spraying sand over the dunes in friendly pursuit. No malice in the chase. Just an amiable drag between young man and rabbit. The rabbit, all haunches and big eyes and follow-the-bouncing-dot cottontail, won. I probably could not outrun a rabbit, either, but at least now I might be willing to try. So, backhandedly (and not too logically), this little episode put me in a new athletic category — with a sturdy, fast-running college boy. Not bad for an ex-obese!

I am the potter, the molder, the shaper.

I can choose whether to flare — or to taper.

As sure as a sculptor who works with a chisel,

I'm forming myself as I bolt, gulp or swizzle.

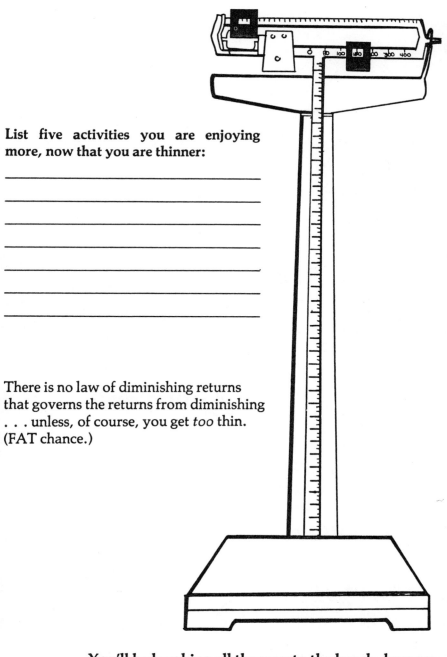

List five activities you are enjoying more, now that you are thinner:

_____

_____

_____

_____

_____

_____

_____

There is no law of diminishing returns that governs the returns from diminishing . . . unless, of course, you get *too* thin. (FAT chance.)

You'll be laughing all the way to the beach, because you are almost at . . .

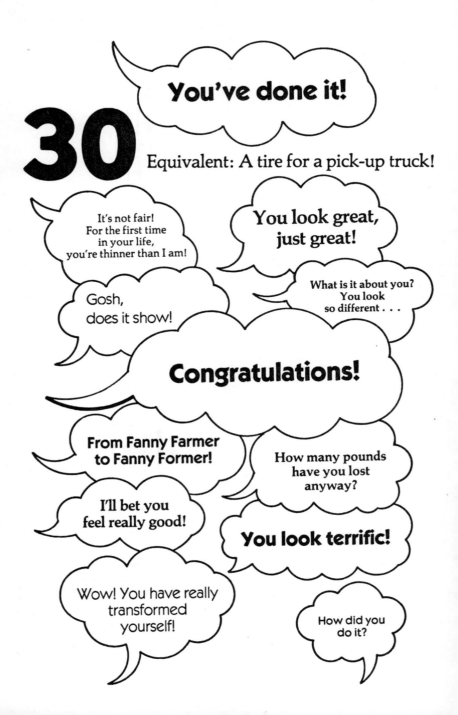

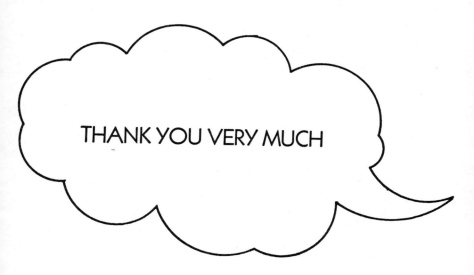

Hooray for me! Hooray for you!

We have done it.

We have freed ourselves from all — or part — of our walls of extraperson. We can be openly, laughingly proud. In the elation of triumph, may we find our balance between "proud" and "smug."

We have not always grinned or hohoed along the course of this thindown. The path has not always been paved smooth by laughter. In fact, we have discovered that the humor which eases anxieties and keeps our attitudes fresh and positive — is also a well-used survival defense that allows us to live in a thin world.

The important thing is — we have learned how to laugh and grow thin.

To my companion thinners:

I have relished your company

May those of us who have not yet arrived at our thinmost keep right on chucking the chub!

The *Laugh It Off* chart follows. Go ahead and copy it for your personal use. Fill it in every day for at least a week. See if it can make you aware of what, when, where and how much — even why — you are eating.

Fill in column one, your eating plan *Layout*, the evening before. The second column, *Any variations*, will tell you whether you are following the plan or deviating from it. If column one and column two do not match, write in your reason for the variation (your pike curled up and burned while you were on the phone, or someone else ate your chicken breast — you arrived as it was being borne away between two halves of a bun).

Column three, *Unusual stresses* is for noting any special anxieties during your day — a family argument, worry over health of a parent or child, an overdue assignment. Under *Good sports*, record both "hidden" exercise (walking to work when you missed the bus, floor-scrubbing, window-washing) and planned exercise (softball with your park team, a spin around the lake on your new roller skates).

How much *Humor* has been part of your day? What did you laugh at? For how long? How many times?

Try to identify your *Immediate* cues to eat — the six o'clock whistle, a phone call at home from your employer, a certain TV commercial. Then pinpoint your eating *Territory*: Where do you eat? In your automobile? In bed? At a cafe counter? On your feet in the kitchen?

Record any *Out-of-the-ordinary* non-exercise activities you engage in beyond your usual job-household realms; mark the activities you enjoy with an E, those you don't enjoy with a D.

The last two columns are reserved for feelings — *Feelings* before you eat, *Feelings* after you eat. Discover whether you are eating as a reaction to certain emotions — anger, hurt, guilt, sadness, joy, relief, anxiety. Can these feelings be traced to your *Unusual stresses* (column three)? Were these feelings alleviated by your *Good sports* or any *Out-of-the-ordinary* activities (columns four and eight)?

This chart does not judge. It is intended only to increase your self-knowledge and to shed light on your eating habits. Unless you have some insights about your behavior, how can you go about changing it?

	L Layout of eating plan (Fill in the evening before)	**A** Any variations: food & liquid consumed NOT on your eating plan	**U** Unusual stresses or anxieties.	**G** Good sports. (Record both "hidden" and organized exercise.)	**H**umo What you la For ho long?
Give Hours					
Morning					
Mid-morning					
Afternoon					
Evening					
After midnight					

Wiggle it off, diet it off, dance it off, wish it

Immediate cues to eat	Territory; where you eat (Be specific)	Out-of-the-ordinary activities. Mark E=enjoy D=did not enjoy	Feelings before you eat	Feelings after you eat

y it off — but get it off

Today's loss:

About the author

Jane Thomas Noland is a free-lance writer and books editor. A former feature writer and editor for the Minneapolis Star-Tribune, she wrote articles about everything from candidates' wives to flower arranging. For twelve years, following her marriage and the onslaught of two children (now grown), she specialized in juvenile book reviews and authored the *Minneapolis Sunday Tribune*'s children's book sections. She is the author of the prayers and "Today I Will Remember" sayings in CompCare Publishers' meditation book *A Day at a Time*, now with nearly a million copies in print. She is co-author with Dennis Nelson of *Young Winners' Way: A Twelve Step Guide for Teenagers* and with cartoonist Ed Fischer of *What's So Funny about Getting Old?* (both from CompCare). Her fiction has been published in *Woman's Day* magazine.

She is a Phi Beta Kappa graduate of Smith College, Northampton, Massachussetts.

She and her husband live in Wayzata, Minnesota.

About the illustrator

Mimi Noland, creator of the well-known hug bears in Kathleen Keating's *The Hug Therapy Book* and *Hug Therapy 2*, also wrote and illustrated *The Hug Therapy Book of Birthdays and Anniversaries*. She is the author/illustrator of *I Never Saw the Sun Rise* (under the pen name Joan Donlan) and the illustrator of *An Elephant in the Living Room, The Children's Book.* (All are from CompCare Publishers.)

She raises pinto sporthorses and ponies and miniature horses on her farm in Maple Plain, Minnesota.

Resources

Alcoholics Anonymous. Third edition. New York: Alcoholics Anonymous World Services, Inc., 1976.

Cousins, Norman. *Anatomy of an Illness.* New York: W. W. Norton and Co., 1979.

Klein, Allen. *The Healing Power of Humor.* Los Angeles: Jeremy P. Tarcher, Inc., 1989.

Lerner, Helene, with Roberta Elins. *Stress Breakers.* Minneapolis: CompCare Publishers, 1985.

Lendon Smith, M.D. *Dr. Lendon Smith's Low-Stress Diet.* New York: McGraw-Hill Book Company, 1985.

Other Books for Weight-Losers from CompCare Publishers

Compulsive Overeater, The Basic Text for Compulsive Overeaters, Bill B. An interpretation of the Twelve Step Program for overeaters by a nationally known speaker. Also includes chapters on abstinence, anger, fear and depression, relationships, money, switching compulsions. 00091, hard cover, 288 pp.

Maintenance, The Twelve Step Way to Ongoing Recovery, Bill B. This companion to Compulsive Overeater helps readers learn to live well, feel good, and maintain weight loss. Highlighted by personal stories of dramatic change and maintained recovery. 00208, hard cover, 352 pp.

The Thin Book, 365 Daily Aids for Fat-free, Guilt-free, Binge-free Living, Jeane Eddy Westin. This weight-losers' classic, with 150,000 copies in print, offers a year's worth of empowering messages that strike at the heart of the problem – sagging motivation. 03046, paperback, 372 pp.

The Thin Book 2, Winning Strategies for All Weight-Losers, Jeane Eddy Westin. A collection of more daily messages about taking charge of your life, weight, and health through key principles of right eating, exercise, and positive attitudes. 03210, paperback, 384 pp.

Thin Is a State of Mind, Nancy Bryan, Ph.D. "Your body is a visible expression of the state of your entire being," Dr. Bryan says. She shows how to tap the power of your "thin mind-set," to begin to remove personal obstacles, relieve stress, and live more serenely – and coincidentally become thin. 03269, paperback, 192 pp.

Write Yourself Thin, Writercizes to Release the Thin Person Within, Toni Lynn Allawatt. A fresh alternative to "diet" books, this applies the therapeutic benefits of journaling to losing weight and maintaining weight loss. A popular workshop leader shows readers how to write their own recipe for forgiveness, see food as body fuel instead of emotional glue, feed appetites with words and images – and more. 04383, paperback, 256 pp.

Order Form

Order No.	Qty.	Title	Author	Unit Cost	Total
04283		Laugh It Off	Noland, J.	$ 9.95	
04383		Write Yourself Thin	Allawatt, T.	$11.95	
00091		Compulsive Overeater	Bill B.	$16.95	
00208		Maintenance	Bill B.	$16.95	
03046		The Thin Book	Westin, J.	$10.95	
03210		The Thin Book 2	Westin, J.	$10.95	
03269		Thin Is a State of Mind	Bryan, N.	$ 9.95	
			Subtotal		
			Shipping and Handling (see below)		
			Add your state's sales tax		
			TOTAL		

CompCare®
Publishers
A Comprehensive Care company

Send check or money order payable to CompCare Publishers. No cash or C.O.D.'s please. Quantity discounts available. Prices subject to change without notice.

SHIPPING/HANDLING CHARGES

Amount of Order	Shipping Charges
$0-$10.00	$2.00
$10.01-$25.00	$3.00
$25.01-$50.00	$3.50
$50.01-$75.00	$5.00

Send book(s) to:

Name _____

Address _____

City _____ State _____ Zip _____

☐ Check enclosed for $_____, payable to CompCare Publishers

☐ Charge to my credit card ☐ Visa ☐ MasterCard ☐ Discover

Account # _____ Exp. date _____

Signature_____Daytime Phone _____

CompCare®
Publishers
A Comprehensive Care company
2415 Annapolis Lane, Plymouth, MN 55441
To order by phone call toll free (800) 328-3330.
In Minnesota (612) 559-4800